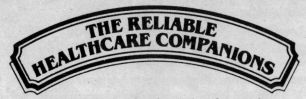

THE RELIABLE
HEALTHCARE COMPANIONS

This book and others in the series
have been prepared to give you a better
understanding of your illness. Armed with the
latest information on all aspects of
ULCERS and other gastrointestinal disorders,
you will be able to minimize the problems
and substantially improve the quality
of your life.

Understanding
—and—
Managing
ULCERS

EDITORS
JOHN L. DECKER, M.D.
AND
PAUL N. MATON, M.D.
THE NATIONAL INSTITUTES OF HEALTH

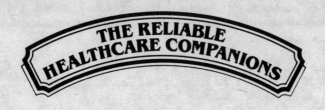

THE RELIABLE
HEALTHCARE COMPANIONS

Understanding
—and—
Managing
ULCERS

EDITORS

JOHN L. DECKER, M.D.
—AND—
PAUL N. MATON, M.D.
THE NATIONAL INSTITUTES OF HEALTH

AVON BOOKS ▲ NEW YORK

The editors would like to thank Hugh Howard, John Gallagher, and Paul Cirincione, whose writing and research assistance helped make this series possible.

THE RELIABLE HEALTHCARE COMPANIONS: UNDERSTANDING AND MANAGING ULCERS is an original publication of Avon Books. This work has never before appeared in book form.

The medical and health procedures contained in this book are based on research recommendations of responsible medical sources. But because each person is unique, the author and publisher *urge the reader to check with his physician before implementing any of them.*

The author and publisher disclaim responsibility for any adverse effects or consequences resulting from the suggestions or the use of any of the preparations or procedures contained herein. No one should ever commence taking drugs or discontinue a prescribed drug regimen without first consulting a physician.

AVON BOOKS
A division of
The Hearst Corporation
105 Madison Avenue
New York, New York 10016

Copyright © 1988 by Gallagher/Howard Associates, Inc.
Published by arrangement with Gallagher/Howard Associates, Inc.
Library of Congress Catalog Card Number: 88-91546
ISBN: 0-380-75428-2

First Avon Books Trade Printing: November 1988

AVON TRADEMARK REG. U.S. PAT. OFF. AND IN OTHER COUNTRIES, MARCA REGISTRADA, HECHO EN U.S.A.

Printed in the U.S.A.

OPM 10 9 8 7 6 5 4 3 2 1

To our teachers and patients alike
this book is dedicated. So often
the two are one and the same.

Table
of
Contents

CONTENTS

A NOTE TO THE READER

There was a time when the physician prescribed in Latin and was likely to respond to a patient's questions with knowing paternalism. ("Now, don't you worry about a thing. That's my job.") Today, healthcare providers—doctors, nurses, and therapists—are beginning to accept the notion that the better informed the patient is, the more likely it is that the patient's condition will improve. There has been, in fact, a clear movement in recent years to harness the patient's curiosity about his or her ailment and put it to use in understanding its nature and treatment. But both patient and doctor face new challenges as a result.

Those doctors who are inclined to educate their patients find themselves so steeped in science and loaded with facts that their explanations often fluctuate between oversimplification and information overload. And those patients who want to be educated have to overcome the comforting notion that the infallible doctor can fix everything. We live in a world where the patient is offered unrealistic hopes of easy cures and instant pain relief by television advertising and media enthusiasm. We have come to believe that there is a harmless pill for every problem and that cures are the norm rather than the exception. While medical science has made incredible progress in understanding the structure and function of living things, there are still innumerable unanswered questions. Sometimes patient and doctor must fact these questions together.

The fact is that, despite the pulsing excitement of research advances, we are today practicing what Dr. Lewis Thomas has called "a halfway technology." We are in a state of mildly confused uncertainty as to what is the preferable choice of action in many medical circumstances. It is this uncertainty, this clangor of divergent advice from many specialties, to which THE RELIABLE HEALTHCARE COMPANIONS Series addresses itself, in the hope that it can enable patients to participate intelligently in decisions about their own medical care.

This book and the others in the series are meant to lead you in your quest for more knowledge, more help, and more support. Your illness may be confusing and, especially in the case of ulcers, its underlying causes likely to be obscure. But we should all understand as much as possible about what is happening to our bodies. By using the resources identified here in conjunction with the guidance offered by your healthcare providers, you should develop a solid foundation for a counterattack at your ailment. I wish you success.

John L. Decker, M.D.
Director, Warren Grant Magnuson Clinical Center
THE NATIONAL INSTITUTES OF HEALTH

PREFACE

Most people confronting a personal health problem like ulcers don't know where to begin.

This healthcare sourcebook differs from the other books on the market in that it is a catalogue of help designed to tell you what to expect of your ailment. Further, this book will enable you to find the kinds of help you need in treating—and learning to live with—your ulcers or your other gastrointestinal difficulties.

Every patient is a unique traveler through the medical landscape. There are no two patients who have the same manifestations, the same course, and the same qualitative and quantitative constellation of accompanying problems. But just as the same map can be given to and used by many travelers, so a sourcebook of help can be given to each person as he or she begins his patient education. You know best your unique problems and concerns; you do not have the same need for information, treatment, and support that your doctor's other patients do; your lifestyle will require unique adjustments that only you can know and make.

But whatever your specific needs, in this book you will find:

- An authoritative yet accessible and comprehensive overview of the problem of ulcers, including answers to your questions regarding physical and emotional management;
- Key information about the role of specialists, community healthcare agencies, and patient support groups;
- Detailed advice on confronting and dealing with the day-to-day concerns of adjusting to the treatment of gastrointestinal disorders through the use of various devices that dispense medication;
- A detailed evaluation of the best available books and other publications about ulcers and gastrointestinal problems;
- A separate and detailed evaluation of audiovisual materials available for rent or purchase;

- Specific advice on how to get access to these kinds of help (800 toll-free numbers, addresses, names).

Increasingly, the medical profession has come to acknowledge the value of patient education. Particularly with a chronic illness, you as an educated patient can, with the cooperation of your doctor, use medication and other therapies and strategies now available to help control your ailment and make it more manageable.

Take advantage of the help in these pages, and of the innumerable sources out there to understand and help your problem: you don't have to fight it alone, nor should you leave it alone.

INTRODUCTION

The statistics relating to ulcers and digestive disorders of the upper gastrointestinal tract are staggering: each year, 1 American in 1,000 develops a stomach ulcer, and over 250,000 are hospitalized with ulcers.

Ten cents of every healthcare dollar is spent for the diagnosis and treatment of ulcers and other disorders of the digestive system. These account for one of every six hospital admissions—more than any other group of disorders. One condition, gallstone disease, affects over 25 million Americans. This year alone, over 500,000 people will have their gallbladder removed, making this the fifth most common operation performed in the United States. The cost to the public? Over $1.5 billion annually.

Unlike some illnesses and diseases that present unique symptoms, many different upper digestive disorders present identical or similar symptoms often involving some degree of pain or discomfort, nausea or vomiting (or both), or change in appetite or weight. Moreoever, the same disorder may affect people differently, producing few, if any, indications of its presence in one case, dramatic signs and symptoms in another. Even when symptoms are present, they do not necessarily correspond to the severity of the underlying problem. For example, heartburn (a common and usually minor digestive problem) is sometimes mistaken for heart attack by the sufferer, while the symptoms of stomach cancer, a very serious disease, are so vague that they often go unnoticed for long periods.

In Chapter 1, we will discuss ulcers and a variety of the other disorders that occur in the upper gastrointestinal (GI) tract. However, in order to understand the various ways in which the GI system fails to function, it is essential to comprehend its normal workings. To that end, the pages immediately following detail the workings of its complex and varied parts.

1

The Digestive System:
How It Works

The meats, vegetables, grains, and other foods we eat contain nutrients, vitamins, and minerals needed by the body in order to grow, replace worn-out tissue, and provide energy for a wide variety of ongoing chemical reactions—in short, the life process. Proteins, essential for bodybuilding and repair, come from sources such as meat and meat products (including milk and cheese), as well as from vegetable sources such as seeds. Fats, a source of energy, also come from meat. A principal source of energy is carbohydrates, which come from plants. Vitamins and minerals from all these sources help the body to work efficiently.

Although food is rich in nutrients, many of these nutrients are not in a form that can be readily used to nourish us. They exist as complex molecules that served the needs of the plants and animals from which they came. Our bodies must first convert them to simpler forms that can be absorbed during the digestive process. Only then can these food constituents be recombined by the body's chemical factory into the complex forms that meet our needs. The function of the digestive system is to move food through the body, to break down the complex molecules into simpler forms as they pass through the system, and to absorb these simpler forms into the body.

What Is the Digestive System?

The digestive system is essentially a tube running from the mouth to the anus, along with various digestive glands and organs including the liver and the pancreas. It is divided into a number of sections, each of which has its own part to play either in the physical and chemical breakdown of food into simpler, more usable forms, in the absorption of these food constituents, or in the movement of food through the system and the expulsion of waste matter from the body.

Much of the digestive process is accomplished by means of powerful digestive enzymes (biological substances that speed up chemical reactions) that assist in the process of breaking food down into molecules small enough to pass through the wall of the small intestines and into the bloodstream.

Once they are in suitable form to pass out of the digestive system and into the blood, the nutrients are transported to all parts of the body. These nutrients ultimately end up as part of the rich liquid that surrounds each cell of the body. Each individual cell uses the nutrients as it needs them, absorbing them through the cell membrane. Once inside the cell, the nutrients are sorted; some provide energy for the cell's activities, others are used to make new tissues or other biological substances such as enzymes.

The Digestive Tract

The mouth receives food, holds it, and helps direct it to the teeth so that it can be torn and chewed into smaller pieces. Proper chewing enables food to be swallowed. In addition, breaking food into smaller pieces exposes more of the food's surface to the action of digestive processes, thereby improving the ability of the digestive juices to work on it.

Three pairs of salivary glands located in the mouth produce saliva, a mixture of mucus and enzymes that provides lubrication and begins the digestive process. An enzyme (called ptyalin) contained in saliva breaks down food and begins to convert it to simpler forms that can be utilized by the body.

The tongue moves the food around the mouth as it is chewed. When the food is ready to be swallowed, the tongue forms it into a small round lump (called a bolus), which it pushes to the back of the mouth and down the passageway that leads to the stomach.

Both the food and drink we take in and swallow (through the mouth), and the air we breathe (through the mouth and nose) share this passageway, but only for a short part of the trip. The passageway branches off: air is carried into one branch of the passageway called the trachea that leads to the lungs, whereas food and liquid is diverted into a second branch called the esophagus that leads to the stomach. To ensure that food doesn't enter the lungs (where it can create an obstruction and lead to a life-threatening emergency), a part of the mouth called the soft palate briefly closes the nasal passages to stop food from entering the back of the nose during swallowing, while another structure, a flaplike appendage called the epiglottis, simultaneously seals the trachea and effectively prevents food and drink from entering the lungs.

In this way, food is carried down the esophagus, and not into the lungs. The esophagus (or gullet, as it is also called) is a muscular tube about ten inches long extending from the back of the throat, through the neck and chest, and finally joining the stomach at the top of the abdomen. As swallowed food slips into the esophagus, waves of rhythmic contractions of the muscle help move the bolus toward the stomach. To reach the stomach, the esophagus passes through a small tear-shaped opening (called the hiatus) in the diaphragm. The diaphragm is a domed sheet of muscle that separates the organs of the chest (heart and lungs) from those of the abdomen.

At its juncture with the stomach, the esophagus has a specialized area of muscle called the lower esophageal sphincter (LES). When food is swallowed, the muscle of the LES relaxes briefly to allow passage of food into the stomach, then quickly closes again. This sphincter is quite effective in preventing the contents of the stomach from reentering the esophagus.

The stomach is a muscular bag located just left of center of the abdomen, just below the rib cage. Its function is to hold, mix, and break up the food into even smaller pieces before allowing it to advance to the next step in the digestive process. When full, the stomach can hold about two and one-half pints of food and has the general shape of a gourd.

Specialized cells (called parietal cells) lining the upper two-thirds of the stomach produce hydrochloric acid. There are approximately 5 million of these acid-secreting cells in the stomach. The acid produced by the parietal cells reduces the bacteria in the food and begins the process of dissolving the solids. It is released directly into the stomach, where it mixes with the swallowed food and salivary enzymes.

Cells in the lower third of the stomach produce intrinsic factor (a substance that allows absorption of vitamin B-12), and gastrin (a hormone that stimulates acid production by the stomach).

Cells throughout the stomach produce mucus, which lubricates and protects the lining of the stomach against the action of the hydrochloric acid.

Another important substance produced by cells throughout the stomach is pepsinogen, which when acted on by the acid becomes pepsin. Pepsin is an enzyme that has the power to split the complex proteins found in food, converting them into smaller fragments.

Precisely how much acid is produced and released into the stomach is determined partly by the food we eat and partly by the action of several different chemicals produced in the stomach and elsewhere. These include histamine, a small molecule that has many important functions; acetylcholine, a chemical messenger released from nerves; and the hormone gastrin. Each of these substances is able to stimulate the parietal cells to produce and secrete acid.

In addition to the chemical action of acid and enzymes, the muscles of the stomach rhythmically churn the food, mixing it thoroughly with the digestive juices.

Generally, food spends an hour to an hour and a half in the stomach, although the quantity and composition of the food you eat has a great deal to do with determining how long a given meal actually remains in the stomach. If the food is high in fat content or has been cooked in fat, its passage may be slowed through the stomach.

Food is partially digested in the stomach into a semiliquid state called chyme, which contains no solid particles larger than a grain of rice. The chyme leaves the stomach as a slow trickle through another muscular ring called the pyloric sphincter and enters the duodenum, the first part of the small intestine.

Cells in the first two inches of the duodenum produce alkali, which helps to neutralize the acid from the stomach. In addition, a substance called bile, which comes from the liver and gallbladder, and pancreatic juice is added to the partly digested food through a duct about four inches beyond the stomach.

The liver, which fills the upper right-hand side of the abdomen behind the lower ribs, is the largest of the internal organs (weighing about three pounds). Considered the body's master factory, the liver has many functions, but its function in digestion is to produce bile, a yellow-green fluid that aids in the digestion of foods by helping dissolve fat. Bile is rich in cholesterol (a fatty substance largely made in the liver), bilirubin (a brown or yellow substance formed by the breakdown of old red blood cells), and various other substances. Bile leaving liver cells trickles through tiny tubes that branch into progressively larger tubes until they form one common duct that empties into the duodenum.

The gallbladder, a small, muscular, pear-shaped bag about three and one-half inches long, is nestled beneath the liver. It serves as a reservoir to collect part of the bile produced by the liver and concentrate it. It can hold about one-twentieth of a pint of bile. When food reaches the intestine, it sends a signal to the gallbladder to contract, and bile is delivered to the duodenum at the time that it is needed.

The pancreas, a gland about the size of an adult's hand, is located behind the stomach. The pancreas serves two different functions. One function is to produce insulin (a hormone best known for its role in diabetes). The other function is to produce digestive enzymes that help break down carbohydrates, proteins, and fats into molecules small enough to be absorbed into the body. These enzymes are carried along with the flow of bile from the liver and the gallbladder before emptying into the duodenum. Like the liver, the pancreas also produces substances that buffer stomach acid and thereby help protect the duodenum from its effects.

The parts of the digestive system discussed so far make up the upper gastrointestinal tract, and disorders affecting these structures are covered in detail in the chapters that follow. Although a discussion of disorders affecting the remainder of the digestive system is outside the scope of this book, its structure and major functions are briefly described here to aid the reader's understanding of the functioning of the system as a whole.

The small intestine, of which the duodenum is the first short part, is the section of the digestive system in which the breakdown of fats, starches, and proteins is completed and the products absorbed. It is a twenty-two-foot-long tube arranged in loops and curls. Many microscopic, fingerlike projections extend into the cavity of the tube and absorb the semiliquid mixture that flows past.

Food entering the intestine is pushed along by waves of contractions of the muscle in the walls. As food slowly makes its way through the intestine, enzymes and other digestive chemicals are constantly working on it, reducing it into smaller and smaller pieces. The muscles of the intestine contract rhythmically to mix the food with digestive juices, enzymes, and bile. These contractions bring digested food in contact with the absorbing surfaces of the intestinal walls. They go on for several hours after eating, and by the time the meal has reached the end of the small intestine, virtually all the food is reduced to molecules small enough to enter the cells lining the small intestine. These cells then transfer the molecules of food to the abundance of tiny blood vessels lining the digestive tract. Once inside the blood supply, these nutrients are transported directly to the liver. Only after passing through the liver are they then free to flow throughout the body to be used where needed.

The large intestine (or colon, as it is also called) connects the small intestine with the anus. Compared to the small intestine, the large intestine is relatively short (approximately five feet long). Food that was not digested in the small intestine passes into the large intestine along with water, generally from three to eight hours after a meal is eaten.

The major function of the colon is to absorb water and mineral salts from digestive products that enter from the small intestine. Approximately one quart of liquid matter enters the colon from the small intestine each day. Most of the usable salts and water are slowly absorbed back into the body, leaving only the indigestible remains of food. This solid waste is called stool or feces. At the extreme lower end of the colon, the rectum stores the waste until a bowel movement occurs and it is discharged from the anus.

The urge to have a bowel movement is often a result of the gastrocolic reflex, a mass movement of the contents of the colon thirty to sixty minutes after eating.

Although the time may vary from between fifteen hours to five days from one person to the next, the average time for the entire process of digestion to be completed is generally about sixty hours.

CHAPTER 1

The Disease

In the following pages, a variety of upper gastrointestinal (GI) disorders are discussed, including gastric and duodenal ulcers and other related and commonplace ailments like gastritis and gallstones. In addition, a number of more obscure but nonetheless important GI ailments are covered.

The discussion of each disorder begins with a list of the characteristic symptoms that would be considered by your doctor in distinguishing one problem from another. In the paragraphs that follow, the nature of the disorder, the likely sufferers, the severity, the long-term effects, and the treatments are described. Disorders affecting the esophagus are discussed first, followed by disorders of the stomach and, finally, disorders affecting the intestine (duodenum), pancreas, and gallbladder.

If your doctor has already identified the kind of GI problem you have, go directly to the relevant section. If you suspect you have a problem, read the symptoms that open each part to help you identify what it is you have. However, you must not rely on this—or any—book to provide you with a diagnosis. That is what your doctor is trained to do. If you suffer from any of the symptoms described, consult your doctor. Proper treatment depends on accurate diagnosis of the underlying problem.

Gastroesophageal Reflux Disease (Reflux Esophagitis, Hiatal Hernia)

SYMPTOMS

- Burning chest pain (heartburn) located behind the breastbone, or vague discomfort in the chest. Usually the pain lasts for many minutes, sometimes as long as two hours or more, and may become worse if the sufferer reclines.
- There may be some difficulty or pain when food is swallowed.
- Symptoms may be most noticeable when the abdomen is under pressure, for example, after meals or when bending, stooping, or straining.
- Occasionally, an individual may become anemic or, rarely, vomit blood.
- Coughing, wheezing, bronchitis, or other respiratory symptoms may develop if, during sleep, the individual inhales acid that has flowed into the esophagus from the stomach.

Gastroesophageal reflux disease is the name given to the signs and symptoms that occur when the delicate lining of the esophagus comes into contact with excessive amounts of stomach juice over a long period of time. The condition may be worsened by irritation due to eating fatty foods, smoking excessively, drinking alcohol, or being overweight. Usually the juice is acid, but alkaline juice containing bile salts and digestive enzymes from the intestines can also wash back into the stomach and then to the esophagus, causing esophagitis.

The esophagus is vulnerable to prolonged contact with stomach juice. When acid comes in contact with these delicate tissues, it stimulates the abundant supply of nerve endings and may cause pain. Strong alcohol or hot liquids may stimulate these same nerves in some people and cause pain. Occasionally, the pain can bear a frightening resemblance to a heart attack.

It is normal for a small amount of gastric juices to reflux (flow backward) into the esophagus (gastroesophageal reflux), provided that it flows back promptly into the stomach. However, prolonged contact of stomach juices with the walls of the esophagus can cause damage to the lining of the esophagus. The resulting inflammation is called reflux esophagitis. In severe cases of acid reflux an esophageal ulcer, or sore, on the lining of the esophagus can result.

Normally, the muscle at the lower end of the esophagus—the lower esophageal sphincter (LES)—limits the amount and frequency with which the acid solution in the stomach enters the esophagus. Sometimes the LES is weak or relaxes inappropriately and allows stomach juice to reflux into the esophagus. At times, these juices may well up (regurgitate) in the throat at the back of the mouth. Acid reflux tends to be worse after big meals and when one lies down after meals or bends over. Weakening of the LES may be caused or worsened by gastroesophageal reflux itself, smoking, fat or chocolate, coffee, menstruation, or pregnancy.

Weakening of the LES increases the likelihood of hiatal hernia (see pages 16–17), which, in turn, makes it easier for digestive juices to enter the esophagus.

The occurrence and severity of esophageal reflux disease depends on LES dysfunction but is also affected by the type and amount of fluid brought up from the stomach, the clearing action of the esophagus, and other factors.

The Typical Sufferer

Gastroesophageal reflux disease is quite common among individuals with hiatal hernia. Since weakening of the lower esophageal sphincter is part of the normal aging process, reflux disease is common among older people. Being overweight or far along in your pregnancy places additional pressures on the lower esophageal sphincter and may also promote the development of reflux disease in some people.

Almost everyone has occasional reflux episodes. Individuals with reflux disease usually have frequent episodes or fail to return the refluxed material to the stomach promptly.

Smoking increases the risk of developing the condition because it relaxes the LES, thereby allowing more refluxed material into the esophagus. Smoking may also directly injure the esophagus, making it less able to resist further damage from contact with material refluxed from the stomach.

Severity

Gastroesophageal reflux disease is a troublesome but not ordinarily serious condition and, with prompt, proper treatment of the underlying cause, rarely results in serious or life-threatening complications. However, prolonged inflammation of the esophagus may cause the development of ulcers and, in some cases, increase the risk of bleeding.

Small quantities of blood passed in the stool may not be readily apparent. Such insidious, long-term bleeding can, however, cause anemia. Laboratory tests performed on a stool specimen can detect such so-called "occult bleeding." In recent years, accurate, low-cost, self-administered tests to detect the presence of blood in stool have been available through pharmacies and drugstores.

Prolonged or severe inflammation may cause sudden and significant bleeding of an esophageal blood vessel, resulting in the appearance of dramatic symptoms. The person may vomit bright red blood or brown blood that has an appearance similar to that of coffee grounds (as a result of the action of digestive juices). If the blood is swallowed, stools may contain liquid blood or have a black, tarry appearance. Whatever form it takes, the appearance of blood is a symptom of a more serious medical problem requiring immediate medical attention. Depending on the duration of the bleeding and the amount of blood loss, the sufferer may experience generalized weakness, faintness, or collapse.

Scarring of the lower esophagus may occur, resulting in a narrowing of the esophagus (stricture), which can seriously interfere with swallowing. If reflux is severe, some material can spill over into the lungs, causing pneumonia or wheezing. Prolonged reflux over years with inflammation of the lining of the esophagus may increase the risk of developing esophageal cancer.

Treatment

For gastroesophageal reflux disease, eat small, frequent meals and try to avoid eating meals late at night near bedtime. Reduce, or preferably avoid, food and drink that you find make symptoms worse, typically such things as fatty foods, chocolate, coffee, alcohol, tomato products, and citrus fruits and beverages.

Avoid wearing tight clothes that increase pressure on the abdomen and diet if you are overweight. Elevating the head of the bed on six-inch blocks uses the effects of gravity to minimize reflux of stomach contents into the esophagus while you sleep. Avoid lying down after eating.

Antacids taken on a regular basis will neutralize stomach acid and reduce the damaging effects of refluxed material, but aspirin should be avoided in all forms. Your doctor may prescribe antacids, acid-suppressing drugs, cholinergics such as bethanechol (Urecholine), motility agents such as metoclopramide (Reglan), or antacids alone or combined with so-called foaming agents, such as alginic acid (Gaviscon), that are believed to form a foam barrier that protects the lining of the esophagus.

Patients who develop strictures of the esophagus may require repeated dilatation of the narrow area, using dilators that are passed through the mouth, into the esophagus, and then withdrawn.

In severe cases of gastroesophageal reflux disease that do not respond to medical therapy or develop complications, surgery may be recommended.

Esophagitis

Esophagitis is an inflammation of the lining of the esophagus. In most cases, esophagitis is the result of the delicate lining of the esophagus coming into contact with excessive amounts of stomach juice over a long period of time. This form of the disorder, called reflux esophagitis, is discussed in the section on gastroesophageal reflux disease (see pages 10–13).

Esophagitis can also occur for reasons other than esophageal reflux. In these somewhat unusual cases, the causes include:

- Drugs, such as tetracycline, potassium chloride, ebepronium bromide (prescribed for bladder problems), and drugs used in cancer chemotherapy;
- Radiation therapy for cancer;
- Infections of the esophagus (such as candida, a yeast infection) that affect persons with poor immune systems, such as diabetics, patients receiving anticancer therapies, and weakened patients taking antibiotics. These conditions allow the yeast to flourish;
- Caustic esophagitis, resulting from household accidents or suicide attempts in which strong acids or alkalis (such as those used in battery acid or drain cleaners, industrial solvents, and other applications) are swallowed.

Esophagitis is occasionally a side effect of a drug or other type of therapy prescribed for an individual's care. Various factors may contribute to the reaction, including the toxicity of the medication and the general state of the individual's health. In some cases, tablets may be swallowed with an insufficient quantity of liquid to ensure that they enter the stomach. As a result, they may remain in the esophagus irritating the delicate tissues with which they are in contact.

The Typical Sufferer

Because of the wide range of drugs that may cause esophagitis in particular individuals, it is extremely difficult to characterize the typical sufferer. However, considering the diseases for which the listed drugs are generally prescribed, it is likely that most individuals who suffer esophagitis as a result of their use are middle-aged or older.

Severity

The severity of esophagitis caused by drugs varies widely. In most cases, it is not a serious condition and, with prompt, proper treatment of the underlying cause, rarely results in serious or life-threatening complications. However, prolonged inflammation of the esophagus may cause the development of ulcers and, in some cases, increased risk of bleeding. Scarring of the esophagus may result in narrowing of the esophagus (stricture), which can seriously interfere with swallowing.

Small quantities of blood passed in the stool may not be readily apparent. Such insidious, long-term bleeding can, however, cause anemia. Prolonged or severe inflammation can cause sudden and significant bleeding or an esophageal blood vessel, resulting in the appearance of dramatic symptoms described in detail elsewhere. (See Gastroesophageal Reflux Disease, pages 10–13.)

Treatment

Treatment of drug-induced esophagitis generally involves changing to another drug better tolerated by the patient, or ensuring that pills or tablets are swallowed with a sufficient quantity of fluid to ensure their prompt entry into the stomach.

Esophagitis due to candida is treated with antifungal drugs, and viral esophagitis with antiviral drugs.

Caustic esophagitis, resulting when lye or strong acid is swallowed, requires immediate admission to a hospital for detailed expert assessment and care.

Hiatal Hernia

SYMPTOMS

- Most people with hiatal hernia have no symptoms and, consequently, are not troubled at all by the condition. Rarely, a particularly large hiatal hernia may produce vague chest pains.
- The burning chest pains often associated with hiatal hernia are, in fact, due to gastro-esophageal reflux disease (see pages 10–13).

A "hernia" is a protrusion of an organ (or part of an organ) through the wall of a cavity in which it is enclosed. In the case of hiatal hernia, the esophagus protrudes at the point where it passes through a natural, tear-shaped opening (the hiatus) in the diaphragm muscle, which the esophagus passes through to connect with the stomach below. A hiatal hernia occurs when the abdominal portion of the esophagus, often along with the upper part of the stomach, protrudes (or herniates) through the hiatus into the chest. This protrusion, or hernia, forms a bell-shaped swelling or pouch at the base of the esophagus in the chest cavity. This can occur if the opening becomes faulty, usually because the muscles and supporting ligaments around the hiatus relax inappropriately or become stretched and weakened.

The Typical Sufferer

Hiatal hernia is quite common among people who are middle-aged or older, especially if they are overweight. Although it may develop at any age and affect either sex, it tends to be more common among women. In fact, the majority of otherwise healthy people past the age of fifty have small hiatal hernias. It may also occur in women during pregnancy as a result of additional pressure placed on the stomach by the developing fetus.

Severity

Hiatal hernias found incidentally do not require treatment and are not medically significant. However, if esophagitis or gastro-esophageal reflux disease is present, treatment becomes necessary. In addition, though rare, a hernia may become strangulated (constricted in such a way as to cut off the blood supply) and may require surgery. Small hiatal hernias are common and usually do not cause symptoms or require treatment.

Treatment

Basically, nothing can be done to make a hiatal hernia go away. If symptoms do develop, they are probably due to gastro-esophageal reflux disease, which can be controlled by medication, modifications in diet, and other measures (see pages 10–13).

If you stuff yourself at meals, you put unnecessary strain on your diaphragm by bloating your stomach. The result may be worsening of a hiatal hernia. Decreasing the volume of food consumed at a meal can be helpful. Eating small, more frequent meals helps minimize the pressure on the stomach.

Achalasia (Cardio-spasm)

Achalasia is a rare disorder in which the muscles of the lower end of the esophagus fail to relax normally, so that food and drink cannot pass freely into the stomach when swallowed. As a result, food accumulates in the esophagus, where it stagnates and serves as a source of chronic inflammation. Although the underlying reasons for the condition are not known, the cause is believed to be an impairment of the nerves that control the muscles of the esophagus.

The Typical Sufferer

Achalasia is most likely to affect individuals who are twenty to forty years of age or older.

Severity

Because it creates a condition of chronic inflammation of the esophagus, achalasia is recognized to be one of the risk factors associated with the development of cancer of the esophagus. When severe, the condition causes weight loss. In addition, particles of food may be inhaled into the lungs during sleep, resulting in pneumonia or a lung abscess.

Treatment

In some cases, a doctor can treat the constriction at the lower end of the esophagus by mechanically stretching the muscles in this area to widen the opening. The doctor does this by passing a slender rubber bag down the esophagus until it reaches the narrowed area, then inflating the bag with water or air to dilate the passageway. In most patients symptoms are sufficiently relieved to allow the individual to eat a normal diet.

In those cases in which mechanical stretching of the esophagus is not helpful, relief from the condition generally requires use of a surgical procedure called cardiomyotomy, in which some of the muscles at the entrance to the stomach are cut to create a larger opening for passage of food from the esophagus.

Cancer of the Esophagus

SYMPTOMS

- Progressive difficulty, discomfort, or, in some cases, pain when food is swallowed. At first, symptoms may appear only occasionally.
- An uncomfortable pressure or feeling of fullness in the esophagus. When swallowing, food may seem to "stick" in the throat. The person may attempt to chew foods more thoroughly before swallowing or may switch to eating softer foods, but the benefit of these efforts, if any, are short-lived.
- Symptoms tend to progress rapidly and become persistent. Difficulties in swallowing soon extend to soft foods and even to liquids. Appetite is severely affected and, as a result, the sufferer may experience rapid and progressive weight loss.
- There may be signs of anemia and, occasionally, indications of blood may be found in mucus that is belched up.
- A cough, bronchitis, or other respiratory symptoms may develop if saliva enters the trachea instead of being able to pass through the esophagus to the stomach.
- In advanced cases, the esophagus may become almost completely blocked, and the tumor spread to other organs.

Cancer of the esophagus is an abnormal growth (also called a tumor) that begins with the appearance of abnormal cells in the lining of the gullet. The cells in this cancerous growth multiply rapidly, causing the passageway to the stomach to become narrowed and constricted. Given sufficient time to develop, these cells invade deeper tissues of the esophagus and spread to lymph nodes and other vital structures nearby. Cancerous cells from the initial tumor may also spread to other areas of the body, where they cause secondary cancerous growths to develop.

The Typical Sufferer

Cancer of the esophagus is often associated with chronic irritation of the gullet. Fortunately, it is a rather rare disease in the United States, though common in some other countries, including China and northern Iran.

Although its cause is still unknown, men are approximately twice as susceptible to this disorder as women. Cancer of the esophagus most commonly affects people fifty years of age or older.

As with other digestive disorders, lifestyle factors appear to heighten the risk of developing esophageal cancer. It is well established, for example, that individuals who have prolonged exposure to irritants such as tobacco smoke or who habitually abuse alcohol are at substantially greater risk for this disease than those who do not.

Achalasia, a disorder in which the muscular contractions involved in swallowing become irregular and uncoordinated (see pages 18–19), is among the recognized risk factors associated with developing cancer of the esophagus more than eightfold.
of developing cancer of the esophagus more than eightfold.

Household accidents or suicide attempts involving the ingestion of corrosive substances such as battery acid, drain cleaners, and the like are likewise associated with an increased incidence of esophageal cancer many years after swallowing the material.

Barrett's esophagus, a change in the cell surface of the lower esophagus resulting from the long-term irritation caused by the reflux of acid from the stomach into the esophagus, also increases the likelihood of developing esophageal cancer.

Severity

Cancer of the esophagus is a very serious disease. The chances of recovery are best if diagnosis and care are provided at a very early stage in the development of the disease. However, even under these favorable conditions, the chances of complete cure are, at best, only fair.

Effective treatment is complicated by the speed with which esophageal cancer develops and spreads to adjoining areas and other parts of the body. Secondary cancerous growths may affect the liver, brain, lungs, or other organs and structures of the body. As a result, only about one person in ten or less survives for five years or more after the condition is first diagnosed.

Treatment

Since early detection and treatment offers the most favorable outcome for sufferers of esophageal cancer, it is essential that a physician be consulted immediately if the occasional or persistent symptoms described here are noted. Even though it is unlikely that a cancerous tumor will be found to be the source of the symptoms, the prudent person is well advised not to risk the possible consequences of delay.

A wide variety of diagnostic tools are available to the physician.(See Into the Laboratory, pages 63–79.)If a diagnosis confirming cancer of the esophagus is made, a decision as to whether to perform surgery to remove the affected part will ordinarily be made as quickly as possible. Depending on the extent of the cancer, the surgeon may decide to remove the cancerous growth or as much of the surrounding tissue as may be necessary to ensure the most favorable outcome for the patient. If surgery is thought not to be appropriate, radiation therapy alone may be used before or after surgery to attempt to destroy remaining cancer cells and retard growth of the lesion. If it becomes entirely impossible to swallow, a tube may be put into the esophagus through the tumor to keep the passageway open.

Acute Gastritis

SYMPTOMS

- Sudden onset of symptoms resembling heartburn and indigestion.
- Mild, generalized stomach distress or an uncomfortable, bloated feeling in the abdomen.
- Pain may be present, ranging from a dull or gnawing pain in the chest to a sharp, burning pain that suggests an ulcer.
- Nausea, abdominal discomfort, poor appetite, and vomiting.
- Gastritis due to virus infections or food poisoning: uncomfortable feeling in the stomach, mild nausea, and one or two episodes of vomiting, followed by loose stools or diarrhea. In more severe cases, repeated vomiting and recurrent attacks of watery diarrhea (occasionally with evidence of blood), abdominal cramps, loss of appetite, dizziness, headache, fever, and extreme weakness.
- Acute gastritis related to the ingestion of corrosive substances may induce burns of the lips, mouth, tongue, and throat. This is a serious, potentially life-threatening emergency requiring immediate medical care.

Acute gastritis is a general term used to indicate an inflammation of the lining of the stomach. It can result from a large number of possible causes, each of which may produce somewhat different symptoms. In general, however, acute gastritis arises from one of three principal causes.

Gastritis is often the result of so-called "lifestyle" factors, such as heavy consumption of alcohol. Another, often more disabling type of acute gastritis is due to an intestinal virus or food poisoning, which almost everyone experiences at some time in their life. Also included in this category is a life-threatening form of acute gastritis, usually associated with household accidents or suicide attempts, that results from the ingestion of strong acids or alkalis, such as those used in battery acid or drain cleaners, or a wide variety of other toxic substances, including industrial solvents, cleaning solutions, or heavy metal salts. Since time is often the essence in these cases, it may not be advisable to attempt to transport the victim to the hospital or doctor's office. Instead, call the rescue squad, police, or other emergency medical services available in your community, read them the label on the container from which the substance came, and follow their directions precisely.

Acute gastritis may also occur as an undesirable side effect of prescribed or over-the-counter drugs, such as aspirin (particularly in large doses), cortisone or other corticosteroids, and various other antiarthritis medicines. In these cases, the drug itself acts as an irritant on the stomach lining.

Finally, gastritis may affect an individual who is severely ill from other causes, typically someone who is already hospitalized or in intensive care. Bleeding or anemia is often the only symptom of this form of gastritis.

The Typical Sufferer

Gastritis is a common condition affecting virtually everyone on an occasional basis. Generally, such cases are relatively mild and short-lived. However, some people seem to be more susceptible to gastric irritation from a variety of sources and are, therefore, more likely to have more frequent bouts of gastric distress.

Severity

Nearly everyone has an occasional, relatively mild attack of gastritis. Usually pain or vomiting caused by gastritis persists for ony a few hours or a day or two. There is virtually no danger of lasting damage to health from occasional bouts of gastritis.

Sometimes, however, especially in cases of acute gastritis due to a virus infection or food poisoning, an extreme case of gastroenteritis (infection involving the lining of the stomach and small intestine) lasts so long that it disables you. Continued vomiting or diarrhea can lead to dehydration through loss of body fluids, depletion of essential body salts, and a dangerous disturbance of the body's chemical balance. Acute gastritis, particularly in children, may be a severe, even life-threatening condition if vomiting or diarrhea results in significant loss of body fluids. This is also true, though to a lesser degree, for the elderly. Consult your physician immediately and treat the situation as an emergency.

Prolonged or severe inflammation of the stomach lining may also cause the development of an acute gastric ulcer or bleeding of the affected area (see pages 25–28).

Treatment

For garden-variety acute gastritis, eat nothing during the first full day of an attack. Instead, drink small amounts of nonalcoholic liquids, preferably milk or water, frequently. After twenty-four hours, begin to eat, but eat only foods you know agree with you, and eat only a little at a time. If your abdominal pain is troublesome, take antacids but avoid aspirin. If you have repeated attacks of gastritis that seem to be related to your intake of alcoholic drinks or tobacco smoke, try to give up drinking or smoking for a month. If this works, the rest is up to you. Certainly, do not burden your stomach with excessively hot or spicy foods or those that provoke attacks.

Frequent bouts of gastritis may be related to your lifestyle. You probably eat, drink, or smoke too much or too carelessly. Once you have found a likely cause and reduced or eliminated it from your lifestyle, you may find that your attacks diminish or disappear entirely.

If your disorder is clearly gastritis, your doctor will probably prescribe an antacid. For severe nausea and vomiting, you may be given an injection of a drug that prevents vomiting. If a drug seems to be causing the gastritis, your physician may advise a change of medication and talk with you about the best timing for taking regular doses.

For acute gastritis due to swallowing of corrosive chemicals, prompt emergency treatment is necessary. Care may include antibiotics, drugs to induce vomiting, and a stomach tube to remove the caustic material.

Acute Gastric/ Duodenal Erosions

SYMPTOMS

- Often, the only symptom is anemia or gastrointestinal bleeding. A small amount of blood may mix with the contents of the stomach and pass undetected in the stool.
- Sudden and significant bleeding may occur if the erosion affects a blood vessel.

An acute gastric or duodenal erosion is a very shallow raw spot (ulcer) that develops in the stomach or duodenum. It is also sometimes called acute stress ulcers. The size is generally quite tiny, a scrapelike sore less than a quarter of an inch in size. In severe cases, a hundred or more of these erosions may be present in an individual.

People with acute gastric or duodenal erosions are often already being treated for severe trauma (such as burns or head injuries), illness or infection, or tumors of the brain. Some individuals may have been taking steroids or large doses of aspirin.

Scientists suspect that the resistance of the lining of the stomach to acid is lowered in individuals who are severely ill or who have suffered trauma; in such people, normal or even lower than normal amounts of acid can lead to the formation of an erosion. It is thought that the lack of resistance of the stomach lining in such cases allows the acid to break down the stomach lining in much the same way that this juice digests food.

The most common causes of acute gastric or duodenal erosions include trauma, which may result from serious burns, automobile accidents, and similar events. Surgery is also a known cause of acute gastric ulcer, particularly surgical procedures that involve the brain.

In addition, it is well known by doctors that a variety of substances, including alcohol, certain drugs, chemicals, and food ingredients, can damage the stomach lining. Among the most common medications known to be associated with acute gastric ulcer is aspirin.

Although aspirin is often considered a relatively safe drug, it is not without side effects, including irritation of the stomach and some degree of interference with the blood's ability to clot. In addition to its widespread use for treatment of headache and other minor pain, aspirin is often recommended for inflammatory disorders such as arthritis. In such cases, as many as twenty-four tablets a day may be prescribed. Although recent medical reports indicate that daily doses of aspirin may be helpful in preventing strokes, daily aspirin doses may have the unanticipated effect of increasing the chances of developing acute gastric or duodenal erosions. Because aspirin also interferes with the clotting properties of blood, the risk of significant bleeding is increased. Further, because headache may be one of the symptoms of upper GI disorders, a sufferer may take aspirin for relief. This can further damage the stomach lining and be the "final straw" that precipitates significant gastrointestinal bleeding.

Similarly, cortisone and other corticosteroid drugs prescribed for the reduction of inflammation common in arthritis and other inflammatory disorders can produce acute gastric or duodenal erosions, but less so than aspirin. The damage produced by any of these causes, in turn, lowers the resistance of the stomach lining to acid and pepsin.

The Typical Sufferer

Since two of the most common causes of acute gastric or duodenal erosions (trauma and surgery) can occur to anyone at any age, ulcers from these factors do not lead to a "typical sufferer."

However, aspirin and corticosteroid drugs related to the treatment of inflammatory disorders such as arthritis are more likely to affect people in middle age or later, with most cases first diagnosed in persons between the ages of fifty and sixty years.

Severity

Acute gastric or duodenal erosions are often accompanied by bleeding, which may be severe. When this occurs in an individual already severely ill from other causes, the combination may prove life-threatening. For example, a significant percentage of people in hospital intensive care units who have kidney failure or infection die from gastrointestinal bleeding due to severe gastritis (see pages 22–24) with numerous stress ulcers in the stomach or duodenum.

Minor bleeding, due to ulceration of the lining of the stomach or duodenum, is quite common. Gradually, if the quantity of blood involved is small, it mixes with the contents of the stomach and passes undetected in the stool. Depending on the extent and duration of such bleeding, it is possible for the affected individual to develop anemia.

However, in some cases, sudden and significant bleeding due to the erosion of a blood vessel may occur, resulting in the appearance of dramatic symptoms. The person may vomit bright red blood or brown blood that has an appearance similar to coffee grounds (as a result of the action of digestive acids). If the blood remains in the digestive tract, the stools may contain liquid blood or have a black, tarry appearance. Whatever form it takes, the appearance of blood is a symptom of a more serious medical problem requiring immediate medical attention. Depending on the duration of the bleeding and the amount of blood loss, the sufferer may experience weakness, faintness, or collapse.

The sudden, brisk bleeding which sometimes occurs can be dangerous, particularly in an older person. The principal danger from bleeding erosions is shock—a life-threatening condition in which the flow of blood throughout the body becomes suddenly inadequate and vital parts, deprived of oxygen, cease to function, at least briefly. When shock develops, the body's condition begins a slippery downward slide. As the brain is affected by the lack of oxygen, the blood vessels swell and become unresponsive because the nervous system cannot control blood vessel diameter as it normally does. The blood pressure then drops even further because the blood vessels are enlarged. Once on this downward slide, the body cannot recover by itself.

There is also a risk that the erosion may perforate the wall of the stomach, although this is rarer than in cases of chronic ulcers. A perforation in the stomach allows the stomach's contents to leak into the abdominal cavity, leading to peritonitis (an inflammation of the tissues lining the organs and inner surface of the abdomen). When this happens, immediate surgery to repair the opening is essential. Perforated ulcer is an unusual, though not excessively rare, cause of death.

Treatment

Acute gastric or duodenal erosions giving rise to bleeding occurring often in otherwise sick individuals require intensive monitoring and support, possibly including blood transfusions, special X rays, drug therapy, and surgery.

Chronic Gastric (Peptic) Ulcer

SYMPTOMS

- Contrary to popular belief, there may be no symptoms, or there may be a dull, burning, gnawing, or cramplike pain throughout the center of the abdomen, or through to the back.
- Pain is usually mild or only moderately severe; it may more closely resemble abdominal soreness or a severe hunger pang than pain.
- Loss of appetite and weight may be present. Nausea or vomiting, distension (an uncomfortable feeling of fullness), or belching may occur.
- Pain or discomfort tends to be episodic, with weeks of intermittent pain alternating with symptom-free periods. Each episode is likely to last anywhere from a half hour to three or more hours.
- Pain or discomfort may develop one to three hours after meals. Approximately one-third of sufferers are awakened from their sleep in the early hours of the morning by stomach distress.
- Severe or agonizing pain may be a sign of a perforated ulcer (see pages 27–28). The affected area over the ulcer will be tender to the touch and the abdomen may feel as hard as a board. Fever and shallow breathing may develop. Perforation of the ulcer is a medical emergency requiring immediate professional care.
- Anemia or minor gastrointestinal bleeding may be noted. A small amount of blood may mix with the contents of the stomach and pass undetected in the stool.
- Sudden and significant bleeding may occur if the ulcer affects a blood vessel.

A chronic gastric ulcer is a raw spot that develops in the stomach. It is also sometimes called a peptic ulcer because of an accident in medical history in which, in addition to stomach acid, the enzyme pepsin was incorrectly believed to be required for its formation. In fact, acid secretion and pepsin secretion always parallel each other. Each can be damaging, but the combination of acid

and pepsin is more damaging than either alone. The size of a
gastric ulcer may vary from a small sore less than a quarter inch
in size to a deep cavity (called an ulcer crater) that may be one
to two inches wide, surrounded by an inflamed area.

Most people with chronic gastric ulcer produce normal, or less
than normal, amounts of stomach acid. In some cases, specifical-
ly those in which the ulcer is near the duodenum, the stomach
may develop an ulcer due to large amounts of acid.

Scientists suspect that the resistance of the stomach lining to
acid is lowered in those people who develop stomach ulcers and
that normal or even less than normal amounts of acid can lead
to the formation of an ulcer. It is thought that the lack of resistance of the stomach lining allows the acid to break down the
stomach lining in much the same way that this juice digests food.
How or why the resistance is lowered is not known. However,
it is likely that a combination of environmental and genetic factors is responsible for this phenomenon.

Some of the same factors that cause acute gastric or duodenal
erosions may also cause chronic ulcers, including the use of cortisone and other corticosteroid drugs taken to relieve arthritis, and
the use of aspirin. The reader should refer to the discussion of
acute gastric or duodenal erosions (pages 25–28).

The Typical Sufferer

In the United States each year, about one person in a thou-
sand develops an ulcer in the lining of the stomach. Although
stomach ulcers can develop in people of any age, they are relatively uncommon in people under forty. In the vast majority of
cases, ulcers are a condition more likely to occur in middle age
or later, with most cases first diagnosed in persons between the
ages of fifty and sixty years. They are more common in men than
women.

Heredity plays a role in the development of some ulcers, although the majority of people with stomach ulcers do not have
a family history of this type of ulcer. However, if a member of

a family develops a stomach ulcer, it is more likely that another close family member will also develop one.

Certain characteristics of the lifestyle of an individual may increase susceptibility to chronic gastric ulcer. These factors include smoking and the use of aspirin or corticosteroids. There is no evidence, however, to support the long-held but erroneous belief that people unable to have regular, unhurried meals are prone to ulcers.

Severity

While ulcers can be a painful and incapacitating condition, they are not in and of themselves a particularly serious medical problem. If they produce abdominal pain or discomfort sufficient to bring you to a doctor, they can be effectively treated and pose little risk of serious consequences. However, lack of symptoms or failure to seek medical care for abdominal distress may allow an ulcer to progress to the point where it can pose potentially serious medical problems.

Failure to detect and treat a gastric ulcer may lead to serious weight loss. This may be due to the effects of poor nutrition caused by reduced eating due to the pain, lack of appetite, or both.

As with acute gastric erosions, chronic gastric ulcers may cause prolonged slow, hidden bleeding or sudden, brisk bleeding that can cause shock. There is also a risk that the ulcer may erode through (perforate) the wall of the stomach. This complication is discussed in detail under acute gastric/duodenal erosions (pages 25-28). In addition, some gastric ulcers are found to be cancerous (see pages 37-39).

Recurrent stomach ulcers may also rarely cause pyloric stenosis, a rare disorder that occurs when the outlet from the stomach (the pylorus) to the duodenum becomes partially or completely blocked. This condition may also be caused by duodenal ulcer or cancer of the stomach (pages 37-45). Scar tissue forms in the passageway between the stomach and the duodenum and forms a block or obstruction to the passage into the lower digestive tract. Whatever the underlying cause, the stomach cannot empty normally into the duodenum. This produces an uncomfortable, swollen abdomen, copious vomiting of previous meals, and foul-smelling gas that is belched up. If the pylorus becomes severely narrowed, repeated vomiting may eventually result in loss of weight, dehydration through loss of body fluids, malnutrition, and a dangerous disturbance in the body's chemical balance.

Treatment

First and foremost, consult your physician when symptoms develop. The symptoms of ulcers are also symptoms of other, more serious conditions. Diagnosis by a physician is essential to ensure that proper treatment is provided.

The symptoms of a stomach ulcer will disappear in about half the cases after six weeks even with no treatment, and the ulcer will heal completely in about two-thirds of the cases in twelve weeks. The old-fashioned treatment of bed rest has been shown recently not to help ulcer healing. Although there is no clear-cut evidence, it seems wise to eat small, frequent meals; take antacids to relieve pain; and avoid smoking, alcohol, and aspirin. Antacid pills in sufficient doses will heal ulcers more quickly.

In addition to these self-help measures, the doctor is likely to prescribe drugs such as cimetidine to reduce the amount of acid produced by the stomach and other drugs to speed the natural healing process. Within six to eight weeks, the ulcer should have healed. Your doctor, in all likelihood, will want to check that it has healed with an X-ray study or endoscopy.

Stomach ulcers commonly recur, some 55 to 90 percent in six to twelve months, especially in heavy smokers. If your symptoms recur, your physician may recommend that you take a regular "maintenance" dose of a prescribed acid-reducing drug at night.

If the ulcer does not heal after twelve to fifteen weeks of drug treatment, or if your recovery is only temporary, surgery may be advisable. Removal of a small portion of the stomach that contains the ulcer will generally eliminate the problem.

Zollinger–Ellison Syndrome

> ### SYMPTOMS
>
> - Severe, multiple ulcers of the duodenum and stomach that are unresponsive to treatment and apparently incurable.
> - All the symptoms of chronic duodenal ulcer (see pages 40–45) may be present.
> - Diarrhea or vomiting may occur whether or not other symptoms of ulcer are present.

Zollinger–Ellison syndrome is a rare digestive disorder in which a gastrin-secreting tumor (gastrinoma) forms in the duodenum or pancreas. The tumor may be malignant (cancerous) or benign (noncancerous).

Gastrin is a hormone (a specialized chemical messenger) normally produced and released by the stomach in response to the entry of food. It stimulates production and release of hydrochloric acid. Normally, as the acid in the stomach rises to a concentration sufficient to digest the food, it acts to inhibit further production and release of gastrin.

In Zollinger–Ellison syndrome, high concentrations of stomach acid fail to exert any regulatory control over the hormone-secreting tumor. As a result, release of the hormone produced by the tumor continues and, in response to its chemical message, the stomach continues to release large amounts of acid.

The coating of mucus and other protective barriers that normally serve to protect the duodenum's delicate lining from the corrosive action of the acid are overwhelmed by excessive acid. Extensive inflammation results, followed by the development of multiple ulcers, most typically in the duodenum. This damage, in turn, further lowers the resistance of the duodenum to both acid and pepsin. In addition, the large amount of acid may impair the function of the small intestine, causing diarrhea.

The Typical Sufferer

Zollinger–Ellison syndrome has no typical sufferer, although one form of the disease does tend to run in families.

Severity

Zollinger–Ellison syndrome can be an extremely serious digestive problem. Because of the extremely high amount of acid produced by the stomach, there are likely to be multiple ulcers. Ulcers tend to develop in unusual sites, and damage is likely to be more severe. There is also a greater likelihood of complications than in cases of common ulcers.

Since multiple ulcers are often involved, it is quite probable that the individual will suffer painful, perhaps incapacitating effects. In addition, there is a far greater likelihood that the serious complications sometimes associated with ulcers, including bleeding, perforation of the digestive tract, and pyloric stenosis, will develop. (See Duodenal [Peptic] Ulcer, pages 40–45.)

In addition, since the symptoms of Zollinger–Ellison syndrome do not respond to the usual doses of medication and other care prescribed for gastric or duodenal ulcer, damage to the stomach and digestive tract may progress until a definitive diagnosis of the condition is made and effective treatment begun. (See Blood Test for Gastrin, pages 72–73.)

Moreover, since Zollinger–Ellison syndrome is caused by a tumor in the pancreas, the tumor itself may also require treatment.

Treatment

Currently, the mainstay of treatment for Zollinger–Ellison syndrome is the use of a class of drugs called H2 blockers (pages 84–85. These drugs (such as ranitidine) suppress the high level of acid production characteristic of the tumor involved. A new drug called omeprazole (pages 90–91) promises to be up to ten times more effective in suppressing acid production than these drugs. Omeprazole is currently undergoing evaluation prior to its release for widespread use. Preliminary studies suggest the drug is well tolerated by patients who have used it. If its long-term safety meets required standards, the drug may soon be available.

Before the H2 blockers were available, the only effective treatment of Zollinger–Ellison syndrome was surgical removal of the whole stomach, which removed the acid but left the tumor, or better, removal of the gastrin-producing tumor. When surgery is an appropriate choice, the procedure usually involves removal of the tumor (performed only in highly specialized medical centers). As with any form of major surgery, these procedures are not without risks, particularly for older patients; those with serious, coexisting conditions such as heart problems or diabetes; and those in a generally weakened state of health.

Atrophic Gastritis

SYMPTOMS

- There may be few or no symptoms, or a vague feeling of abdominal discomfort.
- Undiagnosed atrophic gastritis can lead to a condition called pernicious anemia, which causes fatigue, shortness of breath, and heart palpitations or fluttering, particularly during exertion. The skin may appear pale or yellowed. Other symptoms include difficulty in walking or in maintaining balance, tingling in the hands and feet, depression, mental confusion, and impaired memory.

Atrophic gastritis is a condition, which, as the name suggests, is due to atrophy (a wasting away) of the stomach. The tissue lining the stomach is thinned and the production of essential stomach secretions are reduced significantly in a proportion of the individuals with chronic atrophic gastritis.

One of these substances, the so-called "intrinsic factor," is essential to the absorption of vitamin B-12 in the intestine. Without intrinsic factor, vitamin B-12 deficiency, and subsequent pernicious anemia, develop.

Autoimmune reactions may also be the underlying cause of atrophic gastritis. In these cases, the body's defense system is mobilized, begins to produce antibodies (substances that protect the body against infection), and attempts to destroy the stomach as it would a foreign substance. The process is similar, though not on the same scale, to that of rejection following organ transplantation except, of course, that in this case it is the body's own organ that is under attack.

The Typical Sufferer

Atrophic gastritis is most common in people over sixty-five years of age. In those with pernicious anemia, there may be a history of autoimmune diseases such as lupus, thyroid disease, or certain forms of arthritis. For reasons which are not yet known, pernicious anemia is especially common in blond, blue-eyed persons of Scandinavian descent.

Severity

The vitamin B-12 deficiency associated with this disorder can have severe consequences if not diagnosed and treated promptly. There is a risk of permanent damage to the spinal cord and impairment to intellectual functioning. The risk of developing gastric cancer is increased about threefold in persons with pernicious anemia.

Treatment

If the condition arises as a consequence of the aging process, treatment is largely limited to providing vitamin B-12 by regular injection if needed. These injections will be given by the doctor or, after proper instruction and practice, by the patient himself or a family member. In either case, these injections will be necessary for the balance of the patient's life.

Stomach Cancer

SYMPTOMS

- Initially, there are no symptoms, or symptoms resemble minor indigestion.
- As the disease progresses, one or more indefinite symptoms may be noted, including vague, persistant abdominal pain; indigestion; or an uncomfortable feeling of fullness following meals. Belching, nausea, and occasional vomiting after eating are also common and, in fact, may be seen as the cause of a poor appetite and resulting weight loss. Other early symptoms include pallor and fatigue.
- Symptoms may or may not bear a predictable relationship to meals and may or may not be relieved by food or antacids. The sheer unrelenting persistence of symptoms should alert the sufferer to the possible seriousness of the situation.
- Late symptoms include severe pain in the upper abdomen, difficulty swallowing, frequent vomiting, and, in about 80 percent of cases, a noticeable weight loss. Indications of internal bleeding may be noted, either in the form of bloody vomit (which, as a result of the action of stomach acids, may have the appearance of coffee grounds) or foul-smelling, dark and tarry stools.
- Anemia (a condition in which the number of red blood cells is less than normal) may develop and cause palpitations or breathlessness on exertion, fatigue, and swollen ankles.
- Failure of a stomach ulcer to heal or to stay healed may be indicative of an ulcerating cancer.

Stomach cancer is an abnormal growth (also called a tumor) that commonly begins as an ulcer in the lining of the stomach. Unlike noncancerous (or benign) tumors that also sometimes develop in the stomach, the cells in a cancerous growth multiply and spread uncontrollably. Given sufficient time to develop, they may invade the deeper tissues of the stomach and metastasize (that is, spread) to other areas of the body, where they cause secondary growths.

Unfortunately, the great majority of tumors which form in the stomach prove to be cancerous.

The Typical Sufferer

Stomach cancer is often associated with long-term irritation of the stomach. For this reason, those suffering from chronic gastritis (pages 35–36) are recognized to be at risk for developing stomach cancer. Although the risk is relatively slight, it is a good reason why people with digestive problems should seek the advice of their physicians.

Age is certainly a factor and, though stomach cancer can affect anyone at any age, it is most common in people forty-five or older. The initial diagnosis of stomach cancer is often made in persons between the ages of fifty-five and sixty-five years. Men are more likely to develop the condition than women by a margin of three to two.

Those who smoke run a higher risk of the condition. Heredity also may play a role since people with a family history of stomach cancer appear to have a somewhat higher chance of developing the disease, as do people with blood group A.

As in other digestive disorders, lifestyle factors appear to contribute to the risk of developing stomach cancer. Evidence suggests that a high intake of salt and nitrate increases the chance of developing stomach cancer.

Severity

Although the death rate from stomach cancer has been declining steadily and significantly for almost thirty years, it still remains one of the leading causes of death in the United States.

Complicating the severity of the disease is the fact that, typically, it produces few, if any, symptoms in its early stages of development. This often serves to delay diagnosis and care until the disease has already spread too widely to be stopped.

Once cancerous cells are established within the lining of the stomach, they will invade deeper tissues of the stomach and spread to other areas of the body. Such so-called "secondary" (or metastatic) cancers may affect the lungs, brain, liver, bones, and virtually any other organ or structure of the body.

Treatment

First and foremost, anyone suffering the mild, but persistent, symptoms described earlier should consult their physician as soon as possible. As noted, early detection and prompt treatment offer the best hope for successful care.

If detected at the earliest stage, treatment will involve surgical removal of the cancer and much of the surrounding tissue. A complete cure can be expected in those cases where the cancerous cells affect only the lining of the stomach.

In cases where the cancer has affected deeper tissues or has spread to other areas of the body, the chances of recovery are much less, and treatment may include surgery, radiotherapy, or chemotherapy.

Duodenal (Peptic) Ulcer

SYMPTOMS

- Although there may be no symptoms, most sufferers experience recurrent bouts of abdominal discomfort or dull, gnawing pain, usually localized in a small spot somewhere in the upper middle abdomen or in the back.
- The pain may resemble a severe hunger pang, may occur before meals or more than two hours after eating, and may develop at a particular time of day or awaken the person from a sound sleep in the early hours of the morning. Generally, the pain or discomfort can be relieved by taking over-the-counter antacid tablets, drinking a glass of milk, or eating.
- A feeling of being full or bloated after eating, vomiting, or a sudden filling of the mouth with watery fluid ("water brash").
- Occasionally, the person may vomit bright red blood or brown blood with an appearance similar to coffee grounds (as a result of the action of digestive acids). Stools may contain liquid blood or have a black, tarry appearance.
- Without treatment, symptoms may become almost continuous or may gradually go away.

A duodenal ulcer is a raw spot (or ulceration) that develops in the mucous membrane and underlying structures lining the duodenum, the first part of the small intestine. These ulcers generally develop in the part of the duodenum near the stomach; in fact, the majority occur within the first two inches of the duodenum. The size is small, generally about a half inch wide or less, and, though uncommon, sometimes two or more may develop. Like gastric ulcers, a duodenal ulcer is sometimes referred to as a peptic ulcer.

A duodenal ulcer is caused by gradual erosion (wearing away) of the surface of the duodenum by powerful acid and digestive enzymes released by the stomach. The irritation of the lining which precedes actual formation of the ulcer is often apparent to doctors during examination of individuals experiencing early symptoms of ulcer. The diagnostic term used to describe the characteristic inflammation of the lining at this stage of the process is "duodenitis."

Duodenal ulcer is associated with an abundance or overabundance of stomach acid. The pain of the duodenal ulcer is not simply due to the action of stomach acid on the exposed surface of the ulcer. Some people have ulcers but no pain, whereas others whose ulcers have healed continue to experience pain.

The Typical Sufferer

Duodenal ulcer generally affects a person younger than is typically the case with gastric ulcers. Although duodenal ulcers can occur at any age (a surprising number occur in children ten years of age or younger), they are most likely to develop in young and middle-aged adults, typically between the ages of twenty and forty. Most newly diagnosed cases occur in patients approximately thirty years of age. Only 15 percent of newly diagnosed duodenal ulcers are found in persons over fifty years of age. At every age, they are most likely to occur in people who naturally produce large quantities of stomach acid.

Duodenal ulcers are approximately four times more common than ulcers of the stomach. Current estimates indicate that more than one out of every ten men and one out of twenty-five women will be affected at some time in their lives, though duodenal ulcers may be less common than they were thirty years ago.

Contrary to popular belief, peptic ulcers are not any more prevalent among high-level business executives as a group than, say, university professors or civil servants. Duodenal ulcers affect people of all occupations and all socioeconomic groups.

Smoking has several well-established relationships to duodenal ulcers. Not only are heavy smokers about twice as likely to develop duodenal ulcers than nonsmokers, but their ulcers are less likely to heal than those of nonsmokers. The death rate from ulcers, though quite low, is twice as high for smokers than nonsmokers. Nicotine can inhibit the secretions of the pancreas and reduce these secretions that help neutralize stomach acid.

People with a family history of duodenal ulcer are more likely to develop the condition. There is no evidence linking diet or alcohol to duodenal ulcers, and the role of stress, if any, is controversial.

Severity

Although duodenal ulcers are painful, the risk of severe or permanent damage from complications is low, and the ulcers often disappear in time even if they are left untreated. Less than 20 percent bleed or perforate, and sufferers will be relieved to know that cancer does not develop from a duodenal ulcer.

There can, however, be complications from duodenal ulcers, some of them quite serious. Bleeding is more likely to occur than with a gastric ulcer, and even slight bleeding can result in anemia if it persists. Sudden, heavy bleeding of the sort described in acute gastric or duodenal erosions (see pages 25–28) can also occur and may produce shock, an emergency requiring immediate medical attention.

There is also a risk that the ulcer may erode through the wall of the duodenum, a condition that actually develops in about 5 percent of all duodenal ulcers. Perforation of the duodenum causes sudden, intense pain, sometimes followed by shock and collapse. Any such emergency requires immediate hospitalization.

Perforation of the duodenum allows the contents of the intestinal tract to leak into the abdominal cavity, leading to peritonitis. Peritonitis is an inflammation of the membrane that lines the abdominal cavity, stomach, intestines, and other abdominal organs. When perforation and peritonitis occur, immediate surgery to repair the opening is essential. Although perforated ulcer is an unusual, though not excessively rare, cause of death, it is twenty times more likely to occur as a result of gastric ulcer that duodenal ulcer. Peritonitis always develops when the intestine is perforated.

Peritonitis is marked by very severe, continuous abdominal pain. The pain, which is most severe near the site of the perforation, increases with movement, and the entire abdomen is painful when pressed. Some sufferers become nauseated and vomit and develop a temperature, usually some hours later.

After two or three hours the abdomen may swell but, paradoxically, the pain becomes less severe and less localized. This decrease in pain does not indicate improvement in the condition but, rather, that the situation is worsening and requires immediate emergency medical treatment.

Prompt surgery to correct the underlying cause of the peritoneal inflammation (in this case, perforated ulcer) is generally the only possible treatment. After the patient enters the hospital, the contents of the stomach and intestines may be removed through a long tube passed down the throat through the mouth. Antibiotics and fluids are generally given through the veins to treat the inflammation and prepare the patient for surgery. An incision is made in the abdomen, and the perforation (hole) in the duodenum is repaired. Prospects for complete recovery are excellent.

Another complication which can occur as a result of duodenal ulcer is pyloric stenosis, a relatively rare disorder in which the outlet from the stomach (the pylorus) to the duodenum becomes partially or totally blocked. This condition can result when persistent or recurrent ulcers cause scarring of the duodenum at the narrow point through which partially digested food passes out of the stomach into the duodenum. This condition may also be caused by gastric ulcers and, occasionally, by cancer of the stomach. Whatever the underlying cause, the stomach cannot empty normally into the duodenum. This produces an uncomfortable, swollen abdomen, copious vomiting of previous meals, and foul-smelling gas that is belched up. If the pylorus becomes totally blocked, repeated vomiting may eventually result in loss of weight, dehydration through loss of body fluids, malnutrition, and a dangerous disturbance in the body's chemical balance.

Treatment

Taking over-the-counter antacids to reduce pain and neutralize excessive amounts of stomach acid is often sufficient to cure a minor duodenal ulcer. As with other medicines, antacids may have undesirable side effects. Depending on whether the preparation is formulated with calcium, magnesium, or aluminum (or a combination of these ingredients), the antacid may produce constipation or diarrhea. Further information on factors to consider when selecting antacids is available elsewhere (see pages 81–83), but if you are uncertain regarding the best choice for you, always consult your physician or pharmacist.

You should also be aware that some over-the-counter antacids may contain salt, sugar, or other substances inappropriate to particular patients, for example, diabetics, persons with high blood pressure, or those on restricted diets. Always check the ingredients listed on the package to be sure the antacid does not contain substances inappropriate for your use.

In addition to antacids available in pharmacies, your doctor can prescribe stronger and far more effective medicine to relieve your symptoms and promote healing. Drugs such as H2 blockers (which inhibit acid secretion) and mucosal coating agents (which enhance the protective coating of the duodenal lining) are discussed elsewhere. (See Medication, pages 79–85.) With reasonable care, a duodenal ulcer should be completely healed within six to eight weeks.

During the healing process, abstain from taking aspirin or smoking, and reduce or eliminate your intake of colas and coffee (even decaffeinated coffee can cause discomfort and increase stomach acid secretion). At one time, a generation or so ago, two weeks of bed rest was the recommended treatment. This is probably not effective and, in any case, is impractical for most people.

Contrary to popular belief, ulcers are not treated with a bland diet. In fact, it is not generally necessary to change the foods that are normally in the diet, except, of course, to avoid those that appear to produce or worsen pain. Some sufferers find it helpful to avoid particular foods or drinks, most notably coffee or spicy foods, though each person must determine for himself which, if any, foods are associated with distress. Some sufferers find milk to be helpful in relieving the distress associated with duodenal ulcers. Often, it is the quantity of food, as well as its content, that is likely to be important. Small, frequent meals may be preferred by the sufferer to the traditional three full meals. Food in the stomach tends to neutralize the acid that causes pain. For this reason, many individuals with ulcers eat more or less continuously and, as a result, often gain weight. Missing meals or eating irregularly is likely to worsen symptoms.

For the majority of sufferers, duodenal ulcers recur over a five- to ten-year period, following a characteristic pattern. Typically, periodic bouts increase in frequency and severity, gradually taper off over the course of years, and finally come to an end as the patient gets older.

Once healing is complete, the doctor is likely to recommend a continued regimen of several small, regular meals and no smoking. If symptoms do recur, or if the ulcer does not heal after six to eight weeks of therapy, the doctor may recommend another course of drug treatment and use of a maintenance dose of an acid-reducing drug. In addition, the doctor will probably do a gastrin test (pages 72–73) to see if you have Zollinger–Ellison syndrome (see pages 33–35).

In those patients with particularly severe and persistent ulcers, surgery may be advisable. Removal of a small portion of the stomach (page 88) or cutting the nerves that control acid production (page 87) may be appropriate for eliminating the problem.

Acute Pancreatitis

SYMPTOMS

- Steady, dull, or boring pain in the middle or upper part of the abdomen. In some cases, the pain may be more mild or may resemble the dull, gnawing pain associated with gastric ulcer.
- Pain often begins after consuming a large meal or overindulging in alcohol. In many cases, the abdomen is tender to the touch, and pain may extend to the chest and back. Pain increases gradually over the course of fifteen minutes to an hour before reaching a peak. Moderate or severe nausea and vomiting may accompany the attack.
- In severe cases, the individual may become quite ill with fever and cold, clammy skin and, sometimes, mild jaundice. Rarely, bluish "bruises" may appear on the abdomen a few days after the onset. Symptoms of shock may develop, including weak and shallow breathing, or deep but irregular breathing. Consult your physician immediately if symptoms of shock develop: they may indicate a life-threatening emergency requiring immediate medical care.

Acute pancreatitis is an inflammation of the pancreas in which digestive enzymes produced by the gland enter into the tissues of the gland and the structures around it. Normally, these chemicals are confined to channels which direct them out of the gland into the digestive tract. When these enzymes come into contact with the delicate tissues and inner structures of the pancreas itself, they begin the process of digesting the pancreas. As a result of the corrosive action of these chemicals, severe damage to the pancreas and to the delicate tissues lining nearby sections of the abdominal cavity may occur.

Acute pancreatitis may occur only once and never recur, or the sufferer may develop recurrent episodes called "acute recurrent pancreatitis."

A chronic form of pancreatitis also occurs (see pages 49–51) and resembles the acute form of the disorder in many ways except that, unlike the acute form, chronic pancreatitis causes permanent damage to the pancreas.

The Typical Sufferer

Although acute pancreatitis can affect young people, it is most likely to appear initially in middle age, that is, in people forty years of age or older. It is most likely to affect individuals who have gallstones (see pages 52–55) or other forms of biliary tract disease, conditions that typically arise at this stage of life. Since women are twice as likely as men to develop gallstones, it is not surprising that obstructed enzyme channels due to gallstones is the single largest cause of pancreatitis in women.

Approximately one-third of all cases of acute pancreatitis are due to unknown causes; however, lifestyle is recognized to be a significant risk factor. Alcohol consumption is closely associated with the development of acute pancreatitis, particularly if there is a pattern of alcohol abuse extended over a period of years. In about 80 percent of the cases of acute pancreatitis, the individual has a history of gallstones, heavy alcohol consumption, or both. However, it should be noted that the widely held belief that pancreatitis is always due to alcoholism is a fallacy.

Other less common causes of the acute form of this disorder include abdominal injury, ulcer in the vicinity of the pancreas, certain disorders including hypercalcemia, and the effect of such drugs as corticosteroids, oral contraceptives, and thiazide diuretics (given for high blood pressure and other purposes). Though rare, pancreatitis can also result as a complication of mumps.

Severity

The majority of people who experience acute pancreatitis ultimately recover completely. However, without prompt medical attention, this disorder can be extremely dangerous.

The possibility that a severe episode of acute pancreatitis may produce shock, a life-threatening medical emergency, must be viewed as the gravest danger of this disorder. The prudent person should consult a physician at the first indication of an attack and remain particularly vigilant for any of the warning signs of shock.

Other complications of acute (and acute recurrent) pancreatitis include the possibility of an abscess (pocket of pus) or pseudocyst (pocket of pancreatic juice) forming in or near the pancreas. A fistula, or abnormal opening between organs, also may develop and can have serious consequences. A fistula may develop, for example, between the pancreas and stomach, producing a variety of resultant digestive problems.

Sometimes an attack of acute pancreatitis may be the first indication of chronic pancreatitis, a far more serious illness. Timely medical care is always of paramount importance in this condition.

Treatment

The initial medical treatment for acute pancreatitis is directed at making the patient more comfortable and putting the pancreas at rest, reducing further stimulation for it to produce and release enzymes. The patient's pain is relieved by appropriate medication, and no further food or drink by mouth is permitted. Instead, the patient receives fluids through a tube inserted in a vein to maintain blood volume at normal levels. The patient is monitored carefully to treat promptly any complication that may arise.

Shortly after admission to a hospital, the doctor may empty the stomach of its contents by suction to reduce its fullness and minimize any further stimulation of the pancreas. In addition, the drug atropine may be given to reduce pancreatic enzyme release and help put the pancreas at rest. If any evidence of infection exists, antibiotics may be prescribed.

After an attack of acute pancreatitis, the doctor will perform tests to look for causes. Diagnosis and treatment of the underlying cause of acute pancreatitis is necessary to reduce the likelihood of recurrence of the disorder. If lifestyle factors such as excessive alcohol consumption are involved, the patient undoubtedly will be advised to eliminate alcohol in the future. Although some patients may find this advice difficult to follow, it may be preferable to the possible consequences of severe chronic pancreatitis.

In the acute form of this disorder, surgery is performed only if an abscess or pseudocyst is found to be a complicating problem.

Chronic Pancreatitis

SYMPTOMS

- Steady mild or moderately severe pain in the middle or upper part of the abdomen. The pain may be dull or cramplike.
- Pain often begins twelve to twenty-four hours after consuming a large meal or overindulging in alcohol. Once pain has begun, it is almost invariably made worse by eating or by drinking any beverage containing alcohol.
- In some cases, the abdomen is tender to the touch, and pain may extend to the chest and back. Pain increases gradually over the course of several hours before reaching a peak. Moderate or severe nausea and vomiting may accompany the attacks.
- Some patients develop insidious pain which, over a period of months or years, becomes continuous.
- Chronic pancreatitis is sometimes painless. The principal symptoms are weight loss (due to poor absorption of nutrients), frequent diarrhea, and foul-smelling, pale-looking stools (the color of putty), with or without symptoms of diabetes.

Chronic pancreatitis is an inflammation of the pancreas in which digestive enzymes produced by the gland enter into the tissues of the gland and the structures around it. Normally, these chemicals are confined to channels which direct them out of the gland into the digestive tract. When these enzymes come into contact with the delicate tissues and inner structures of the pancreas itself, they begin the process of digesting them. As a result of the corrosive action of these chemicals, severe damage to the pancreas and to the delicate tissues lining nearby sections of the abdominal cavity may occur.

In the chronic form of this disorder, recovery between successive bouts is not complete and, as a result, each new episode worsens earlier damage done to the pancreas. Ultimately, the pancreas may be so severely affected that it is no longer able to function normally.

The Typical Sufferer

Although chronic pancreatitis can affect young people, it is most likely to appear initially in middle age, that is, in people forty years of age or older.

Approximately one-third of all cases of chronic pancreatitis are due to unknown causes; however, lifestyle is recognized to be a significant risk factor in the chronic form of this disorder. Alcohol consumption is closely associated with the development of chronic pancreatitis, particularly if there is a pattern of alcohol abuse extended over a period of years.

Other, less common causes of the chronic form of this disorder include abdominal injury, certain disorders including hyperparathyroidism, and various hereditary forms.

Severity

Chronic pancreatitis is a serious condition that can have a major impact on an individual's life, depending on the degree to which the organ's ability to function normally has been impaired.

If the pancreas is no longer able to produce sufficient quantities of the enzymes needed for normal digestion, some degree of disturbance to the digestive process may occur, with resultant malabsorption of food and weight loss.

Similarly, if the insulin-producing cells of the pancreas are damaged extensively, the organ may be unable to provide the body with sufficient quantities of this essential hormone. Insulin affects the body's metabolism, that is, its ability to utilize food. Without it, the body is unable to utilize glucose, the major source of energy that fuels the normal activities of all living cells. As a result, diabetes, a serious chronic disease, will develop. Patients with severe chronic pancreatitis may require daily insulin supplementation in order to live a reasonably normal life. Furthermore, the severe, unrelenting pain may make normal life virtually impossible.

Treatment

The initial medical treatment for chronic pancreatitis is directed at easing pain and stopping alcohol consumption. Painkilling drugs may be prescribed to bring relief to sufferers of chronic pancreatitis, but they should be used very cautiously since they present the considerable risk that the individual may ultimately become dependent on them.

If the patient is admitted to the hospital with an acute attack of pain, he or she will be treated as for acute pancreatitis (see pages 46–49).

Diagnosis and treatment of the underlying cause of chronic pancreatitis is necessary to prevent or reduce further damage to the pancreas. If lifestyle factors such as excessive alcohol consumption are involved, the patient undoubtedly will be advised to eliminate alcohol in the future. Although some patients may find this advice difficult to follow, it may be preferable to the possible consequences of severe chronic pancreatitis.

Good nutrition should be maintained with vitamin supplements if necessary, appropriate control of the diabetes, and ingestion of tablets containing pancreatic enzymes to aid digestion of food. The severe pain of chronic pancreatitis, if due to alcohol, can sometimes be relieved by high doses of pancreatic digestive hormones.

Surgery is considered if pain cannot be controlled by medical means. In some cases in which impaired drainage of the pancreas causes, or contributes to, severe, continuous pain, surgery may be performed to allow the gland to drain into the intestine. The success of this surgery is, however, somewhat problematic and, as a result, the surgery may or may not achieve its objective.

Surgery may also be undertaken if an abscess (pocket of pus) or pseudocyst (pocket of pancreatic juice) is found to be present.

Gallstones, Biliary Colic, and Chronic Cholecystitis

SYMPTOMS

- Many people have gallstones but do not have any symptoms. Because they produce no symptoms, such gallstones are said to be "silent."
- Attacks of biliary colic are characterized by severe, persistent pain in the upper abdomen, lasting from about a half hour to three hours or more. Pain may be felt in the back between the shoulder blades. Some sufferers experience nausea or vomiting.
- Vague abdominal complaints such as bloating, fullness, burning sensations in the stomach, or intolerance to fatty foods.

As previously mentioned, the basic function of the gallbladder is to store and concentrate bile produced by the liver. If the bile is too high in cholesterol relative to other constituents, the gallbladder sometimes produces a solid lump of material called a "gallstone." The most common type of gallstones are composed almost entirely of cholesterol, a substance manufactured by the liver. (In fairness to this much-maligned chemical, associated in the minds of many with heart attack and stroke, it should be noted that cholesterol is a normal constituent of bile and, moreover, is essential in making and maintaining all cells and in producing hormones.) In another, less common variety of gallstone, calcium is the principal constituent.

Although in many individuals these stones cause no problems (and are, therefore, called "silent gallstones"), in many patients they do. Such stones form in the gallbladder, and may stay there or pass out of that organ through the cystic duct into the common bile duct, and then enter the duodenum. For purposes of clarity, it should be stressed that inflammation of the gallbladder is a result, rather than cause, of the gallstone.

Sometimes, however, a stone will become lodged in the small cystic duct emptying the gallbladder, leading to acute cholecystitis (see pages 56–57). It can also lodge in the larger common duct which carries bile from the liver to the duodenum. Complete blockage of this duct causes jaundice to develop. The intense pain experienced by sufferers of this condition is biliary colic. Such patients may also develop infection or acute pancreatitis (see pages 46–49).

If the stone falls back into the gallbladder or is forced along the duct until it reaches the duodenum, the blockage that had been causing the problem is gone and the pain will cease. However, most patients will have been admitted to hospital and will require further tests and treatment.

The Typical Sufferer

Current estimates suggest that as many as 25 million people in the United States (approximately one out of every ten) have gallstones and, it should be noted, most are unaware of it.

The likelihood of developing gallstones is a function of both age and sex. While young people are rarely affected with gallstones, it is estimated that one out of every five elderly Americans has the condition. For reasons not yet understood, women are more than twice as likely to develop gallstones than men, with half those over forty affected.

Excess weight appears to increase the risk of developing gallstones for both men and women, although medical statistics clearly indicate that women who are overweight are at greatest risk for developing gallstones.

Native American Indians, both men and women, have by far the highest incidence of gallbladder disease of any group in the country, suggesting that heredity, environment, or both play a significant, though not yet fully understood, role in the development of this condition. Native American Indian women are particularly susceptible, with studies in some tribes indicating that three out of four women over age thirty already show evidence of gallstones.

In the next year, more than a million new cases of gallbladder disease will be diagnosed in the United States.

Severity

If a gallstone remains lodged in the cystic duct for any length of time, it may block the exit for bile. Inflammation or infection of the gallbladder may result. (See Acute Cholecystitis, pages 56–57.)

In addition, the cumulative effect of repeated insults to the gallbladder can be quite serious. Each time a stone obstructs the gallbladder, there is a new possibility that inflammation and infection will occur. As a result, the gallbladder may become so scarred that it is unable to perform its normal functions (chronic cholecystitis).

Gallstones can also enter and block the channel that drains the liver (the common bile duct). This somewhat less common complication is called common bile duct obstruction. The inability of bile to flow freely from the liver may lead to jaundice, a yellowing of the skin and whites of the eyes due to the presence of the yellowish bile pigment. Similarly, gallstones can block the main channel that drains the pancreas, and cause acute pancreatitis (pages 46–49).

In rare cases, cancer of the gallbladder develops in a gallbladder containing gallstones.

Treatment

Currently, the only definitive treatment for symptomatic patients is surgery, at which the gallbladder is removed. Prior to surgery, most patients will have had an ultrasound examination (see pages 70–71) or a cholecystogram (see pages 78–79). Patients who are thought to have stones in the common bile duct may also require endoscopic retrograde cholangiography and pancreatography (ERCP) (see pages 73–75), or percutaneous transhepatic cholangiography (see page 77).

Until recently, there were no medicines or nonsurgical medical procedures that could dissolve or otherwise eliminate gallstones. However, in the early 1980s, the drug chenodeoxycholic acid (and, more recently, ursodeoxycholic acid) was found to be effective in dissolving stones in patients who are thin and have small cholesterol stones. Although a promising step, these drugs are far from a panacea for gallstone sufferers. In addition to the fact that it is not equally effective for all patients, chenodeoxycholic acid has side effects (including diarrhea and the possibility of liver damage), so it cannot be used in many individuals. Moreover, once the drug is stopped, gallstones may once again develop. The newer drug, ursodeoxycholic acid, produces less of these undesirable side effects. However, it is likely that until further advances along these lines are made, most patients will continue to receive more traditional forms of care.

The success of lithotripsy, a technique in which ultrasound shock waves are used to break up kidney stones painlessly, has prompted research into the possible application of a similar technique for treatment of gallstones. Early indications seem promising despite the fact that it has proven to be more difficult to focus the sound waves properly and, in addition, gallstones do not break up as easily as kidney stones. In those cases in which the technique has been used successfully to break up the stones, patients are then given chenodeoxycholic acid to dissolve the small fragments.

Acute Cholecystitis

SYMPTOMS

- Sudden, moderate or intense, steady pain in the upper right side of the abdomen, usually on the right-hand side, together with tenderness.
- Pain may radiate to the shoulder, shoulder blade, or back. An acute attack often begins an hour or so after eating, particularly if the meal has included fried or fatty foods. Pain may awaken the sufferer from a sound sleep. Generally, the pain worsens over the course of several hours.
- As the condition progresses, the person may sweat profusely and experience chills, pain when the abdomen is touched, nausea, vomiting, extreme restlessness, and onset of fever. Unlike ulcers, the pain of cholecystitis is not relieved by food or antacids.
- Mild jaundice (a yellowing of the skin and whites of the eyes) may develop within a day or so.

Acute cholecystitis is an inflammation of the gallbladder. Most commonly, it results when a gallstone formed in the gallbladder makes its way into the narrow duct that carries bile out of the gallbladder (the cystic duct) and creates a blockage. It is a relatively common complication of gallbladder disease.

If a gallstone remains lodged in the cystic duct for any length of time, it may block the exit for bile. Acute cholecystitis may result.

The Typical Sufferer

People with gallstones are at the highest risk for developing acute cholecystitis. The typical sufferer has had gallstones (often without symptoms of any kind) for a prolonged period, perhaps ten years or more. For a description of the risk factors associated with development of gallstones, see the section on biliary colic and gallstones (pages 52–55).

Severity

Because the pain from acute cholecystitis is generally quite severe, most people who suffer an attack consult their physician or seek care at a hospital. The gallbladder may become so inflamed that it begins to leak bile, leading to a particularly severe form of peritonitis, an infection of the membrane that lines the abdominal cavity, stomach, intestines, and other abdominal organs.

Even though gallbladder disease is not usually fatal, its complications are the cause of death for nearly 6,000 people annually in the United States.

Treatment

A person suffering an attack of acute cholecystitis should be admitted to hospital, given drugs to give relief from the pain, intravenous fluids, and other care. Surgical removal of the gallbladder (a procedure called cholecystectomy) is often recommended at that time or a few weeks later as the preferred course of treatment for patients who develop cholecystitis and other serious complications of gallbladder disease, in order to prevent further attacks or complications.

With more than a million new cases of gallbladder disease diagnosed in the United States each year, it is not surprising that cholecystectomy should rank fifth among the most common surgical procedures performed. Approximately half a million of these operations are performed annually in hospitals around the country.

Functional Digestive Disorders

SYMPTOMS

- Cramplike spasmodic pain in the abdomen.
- An uncomfortable feeling of fullness, belching, the need to pass gas frequently, heartburn, nausea, vomiting, and headache.
- Intermittent bouts of diarrhea, constipation, or alternating episodes of both. Bowel movements often provide relief from cramps.
- Symptoms tend to recur periodically, lasting days or weeks on each occasion, sometimes even longer. This pattern may continue, more or less unchanged, over a period of many years.

Functional digestive disorders are those in which careful examination reveals no sign of disease in the digestive tract. That is to say that the cause of the disorder is not known. Some physicians believe that these disorders may be due to disorders of muscles or nerves in the gut, while others believe them to be psychological. These conditions are not necessarily disorders of the upper intestinal tract but often produce many of the same symptoms as ulcers. They take a variety of forms and affect millions of people annually in the United States.

In all likelihood, there are many such conditions, some of which may include problems of intestinal motility (the waves of muscular contractions that move materials through the intestine), rather than disease or structural abnormality. Included among the conditions often diagnosed as functional digestive disorders are functional abdominal pain, irritable bowel syndrome, spastic colon, mucous colitis, and postcholecystectomy syndrome. Functional digestive disorders are often only diagnosed after X rays and other diagnostic tests have eliminated all other likely causes.

The Typical Sufferer

The recurrent symptoms of functional digestive disorders affect up to three out of four people at some time in their lives. Although the characteristic pattern of symptoms may develop in early adulthood, it is more common in people thirty and over. For reasons not understood, women are twice as likely as men to be sufferers of functional digestive disorders.

Severity

Functional digestive disorders pose no serious threat to health, have no medical complications, and do not lead to more serious disease. They can, and often do, however, make life miserable for those who suffer from them.

Treatment

The doctor may prescribe medications for relief of symptomatic constipation and diarrhea. Sufferers are also often helped by careful attention to their diet, including avoiding foods which seem to bring on symptoms. Others find that a bland diet, or one high in fiber, is best for them. It is entirely possible that, in some cases, functional digestive disorders are in fact due to an underlying food allergy. Some find relief by abstaining from tobacco, coffee, or alcohol.

Stress may be an important precipitating factor for some people and not at all relevant for others. Effective self-help techniques of stress management are available in many pamphlets and books. The effectiveness of these techniques seem to vary widely from one person to the next. If functional abdominal pain is believed to be associated with stress, sedatives may be prescribed. Some studies suggest psychiatric therapy is helpful to some sufferers.

CHAPTER 2

Care and Treatment

Dramatic progress has been made in understanding the causes and care of digestive disorders since prehistoric man first spent a sleepless night helplessly seeking relief from pain that wracked his innards.

The subject of this chapter is the care and treatment of today's sufferer of upper gastrointestinal disorders. In the previous chapter, a number of treatments were referred to in the context of discussing specific disorders, but here we will describe them in more detail. Some of these conditions are acute: with prompt and proper care, the sufferer of a disorder such as acute gastric ulcer can look forward to a complete cure. Some conditions are chronic: the sufferer of a disorder such as chronic pancreatitis may have to live with recurrent attacks for the rest of his life. While the patient with acute gastric ulcer can reasonably expect that medication and attention to lifestyle factors will solve the problem, the patient with pernicious anemia will require regular injections of vitamin B-12 for as long as he or she lives.

Perhaps most important, however, is the fact that unlike the unique symptoms of some disorders that make diagnosis of the underlying problem almost a foregone conclusion (as, for example, "excessive thirst + frequent urination = diabetes"), digestive disorders may lack symptoms entirely or may share many of the same ones characteristic of a dozen or more different conditions.

It is precisely because so many of these disorders cause similar symptoms and because any one symptom could be associated with one of the many digestive disorders that make diagnosis and care by a physician essential.

Determining the exact course of care and treatment for a person with a gastrointestinal problem should be the result of a collaborative effort between you, the patient, and your doctor. The first key step in the process, then, is finding the right professional guidance.

Selecting
a
Doctor

Living with the symptoms of an upper gastrointestinal disorder without a doctor is like driving a car without knowing how. It can be done, of course, but the risks are great.

We already have seen that there are a variety of ways we can be affected by these disorders, some of them serious or potentially so. To make matters more complicated, each digestive disorder may affect sufferers somewhat differently. A good doctor is crucial for determining the underlying cause of your symptoms and devising a suitable treatment program.

As the rest of this chapter points out, there are a variety of treatments possible. Some are as simple as avoiding foods that don't agree with you, using over-the-counter antacids, and reducing the intake of alcohol and other irritating substances. Others involve sophisticated diagnostic tests, surgery, and more unusual therapeutic approaches. But negotiating the tricky terrain of the medical landscape requires a tour guide. Enter your family physician.

The best place to begin dealing with your gastrointestinal symptoms is with a doctor who knows you. Make an appointment to see him or her immediately if you think you have a problem of the digestive system. If your symptoms include persistent, severe pain, a rigid, boardlike abdomen, or indications of blood (either in vomit or stool), get an appointment today.

In Chapter 3 we will discuss the specialists and when they are to be consulted. However, in many problems of the digestive system, such as the "garden-variety" peptic ulcer, the expenditure of time and money to visit a specialist may not be necessary. Instead, it is your family doctor who can provide you with the guidance and treatment you need.

If you have no regular physician, ask your friends or relatives for a recommendation. A local medical society, medical school, or accredited hospital may also be able to help you find a suitable doctor.

If your digestive disorder does not seem to respond as it should to the treatments your doctor gives you, or if you have one of the less common varieties, your doctor may suggest you consult a gastroenterologist, a specialist in digestive disorders, including ulcers and many other conditions. If your gastroenterologist in turn deems surgery to be the answer to one or more of your digestive problems, he or she will refer you to a surgeon.

Into the Laboratory

The symptoms you describe to your doctor (so-called "presenting symptoms") may eliminate some disorders as likely causes of your problem and focus suspicion on others. The answers you provide to your doctor's questions may help narrow the focus of suspicion still further, but, in all likelihood, it will be necessary to conduct one or more tests before a definitive diagnosis can be made.

The test (or combination of tests) used makes it possible to assemble the information needed to identify the condition (or combination of conditions) responsible for your symptoms so that appropriate treatment can be begun.

There are literally dozens of diagnostic tests appropriate for use in particular circumstances. Your doctor will select those most appropriate in your case. The tests identified and discussed in the following pages are among those most commonly used.

The application of advanced technology to the diagnosis of illness and disease has made some tests commonly used only a few years ago all but obsolete. This trend is likely to continue for the foreseeable future.

Upper GI (Gastrointestinal) Series

The upper GI series is one of the most widely used diagnostic tests. The test, as the name suggests, is used to help the doctor detect and identify abnormalities or disease processes in the upper portion of the digestive tract, that is, the esophagus and mouth.

An upper GI series utilizes X rays to help the doctor visualize the internal organs of the digestive tract. If you have ever seen an X ray (which resembles a photographic negative), you know that bones and other dense objects show up clear and sharp, while the soft tissues of the body appear as vague shapes and shadows. Since the structures the doctor wants to view are of this "soft" variety, other steps must be taken to make them stand out clearly for careful visual examination. The technical name for such substances (there are several in common use) is a "contrast agent." Because these tests make use of such substances, they are called "contrast studies."

The contrast medium used in the upper GI series is barium, a powder that is mixed with liquid. When swallowed, the barium mixture fills the hollow digestive tract and makes it stand out in clear detail during the GI series.

To obtain the best results, it is important that the digestive tract be empty of all food at the time of the test. In preparation, the doctor will ask you to refrain from all food and drinks after the evening meal on the day before the test is scheduled.

Just before the test is to begin, you will be instructed to drink the liquid barium mixture (called a "barium meal"). The barium mixture is thick in consistency, rather like a milk shake, and has a mild, though somewhat chalky, taste. It is likely to be flavored to taste like strawberry or something similarly pleasant.

As the liquid passes down the esophagus and into the stomach, the doctor will watch its progress with the aid of an X-ray device called a fluoroscope. Unlike an X ray, which provides results comparable to a still picture, the fluoroscope allows the doctor to have a continuous view of the passage of the barium mixture through the system. At any point in the process at which the doctor wants to preserve particular visual information, a conventional X-ray picture can be taken.

As the test proceeds, the doctor may ask you to move and to assume various positions to improve the view of what is going on. If it is necessary to get an even sharper image, powders or pills that release gas in the stomach may be given. These are often helpful in viewing such details as the surface of the digestive tract. Similarly, if the doctor wants to relax the stomach and open the pylorus (the opening into the intestinal tract), you may be given a small injection of medication.

No special steps are necessary after the test is completed to cleanse your system of the barium liquid; it will be excreted as part of your normal digestive process, generally within eighteen hours or so. To further facilitate the process, the doctor may suggest that you drink extra liquids, particularly if you tend to be constipated.

The results of the test are determined by visual inspection of the X-ray pictures (or "plates" as they are also called). Through training and extensive experience, the physician knows the appearance of a normal, healthy digestive tract, as well as the appearance of the various abnormalities which may affect it. Results are not usually known (or given) immediately after the tests are completed. The doctor who examines the X rays will want an opportunity to study them carefully and present the findings to your doctor. It is your doctor who will then discuss the test results with you.

Because it utilizes X rays, there is some slight risk associated with the upper GI series. X rays are a form of radiation that causes some degree of damage to the body; the greater the exposure, the greater the damage. The fluoroscope, which uses continuous X rays, gives patients a far higher dose of radiation than the standard X-ray machine. Moreover, damage from X rays is cumulative over a period of years and poses particular dangers to young children, adolescent girls whose breasts are developing, and pregnant women.

While the benefits of these tests usually far outweigh the risks, for your protection it is important to discuss with the doctor any and all exposure that you have had to radiation, including earlier X rays. This simple step can help assure that risks are maintained at an acceptable level.

Endoscopy

Endoscopy is a diagnostic procedure that gives the gastroenterologist a direct view of the upper digestive tract from within the body itself. By means of an instrument called a fiber-optic endoscope, the doctor is able to illuminate and follow the same path that food takes, examining the esophagus, stomach, and duodenum from within.

Along the way, the doctor can pause to look closely at inflamed, ulcerated, or infected areas; growths and malformations; sources of bleeding; in short, anything of particular interest. Areas that may appear only as shadowy shapes on X rays and sonograms are seen close up and in living color with the endoscope. Given the detail and accuracy of the information it provides, it is not surprising that the endoscope is one of the gastroenterologist's most important tools.

Fiber optics, as the name implies, are long, threadlike filaments of glass, which, because of their extreme thinness, are also extremely flexible. Hundreds of these fibers are bound together to form a bundle nearly as flexible as the individual fibers of which it is comprised. Most important, the images of objects at one end can be seen clearly at the other, making it possible to look around corners.

The fiber-optic endoscope is fitted with an eyepiece and appropriate lens that provides a magnified view of specific structures, allowing the doctor to examine them close up. With the addition of a tiny self-contained light to provide necessary illumination, the fiber-optic endoscope is almost the ideal instrument for following the twists and turns of the digestive system.

The fiber-optic endoscope, however, is far more than an optical instrument for passive viewing. Designed with internal channels that can accommodate instruments, the same tube that carries the visual image can enable the doctor to collect tissue samples for microscopic examination by a laboratory; remove polyps and other growths; find and stop the source of gastrointestinal bleeding; suction out material; or pump in air to open and extend passages or water to clean the lens or wash the field of view. A permanent record of everything seen can be preserved for further study or comparison to later tests by means of still photographs or videos taken through the endoscope.

At the time endoscopic examination is scheduled, a sample of blood will be taken to check, among other things, the time it takes to clot. This information allows the doctor to prepare in advance in the unlikely case that problems develop during the procedure.

To obtain the best results, it is important that the digestive tract be empty of all food at the time of the test. In preparation, the doctor will request that you refrain from all food and drink for approximately eight hours prior to the test.

When you arrive at the doctor's office or hospital where the test is to be conducted, you will be given a consent form to read and sign. Signing this form means that, before giving your consent for the procedure to be performed, you have been informed by the doctor of the details of what is to be done and advised of any risks that it may entail. Before signing the form, you should take this opportunity to make the doctors aware of allergies and other aspects of your medical history and get answers to any questions you may have. Fiber-optic endoscopy, although safe, is not without risk: unexpected bleeding, perforation of the tract, and other complications can result. To minimize these risks, the procedure should be performed by a properly licensed, board-certified (or board-eligible) gastroenterologist.

Shortly before the test is to begin you will be given an injection of medication to relax you and reduce any discomfort you might feel at the start of the procedure. A line placed in a vein in your arm at this time enables the doctor to administer additional doses of these and other medications that may be required as the procedure progresses. Then the throat is numbed, usually by an anesthetic spray, to ease any discomfort when the endoscope is swallowed and also to reduce the gag reflex which is normally triggered when the back of the tongue is touched. Commonly, a device is placed in the mouth for the mutual protection of both teeth and instrument. With preparations complete, room lights are dimmed to ensure optimal viewing conditions, and the test is begun.

The patient swallows the lubricated tip of the instrument which, having entered the esophagus, is then slowly and carefully advanced under the doctor's control through the digestive tract. While few patients find the procedure pleasant, most tolerate it quite well.

As the test progresses, you may experience nausea or mild cramps as the tube is threaded through your system. Pain and discomfort, if any, can be quickly relieved by the administration of additional medication through the line placed in your arm. The doctor may also introduce medication to stimulate various digestive activities in order that they can be observed. During the test, the doctor may ask that you change position on the examining table. Though sedated and relaxed, you should still be sufficiently alert to follow the doctor's instructions.

During endoscopy, the doctor may take a tissue biopsy. This is a procedure by which a sample of tissue is removed from the body so it can be submitted for preparation and analysis by a laboratory. A biopsy is essential in every case in which the doctor has a suspicion that a growth or other abnormal tissue may be cancerous and wants the tissue analyzed. The findings of such an analysis are, of course, of great importance in determining proper care. In some cases, biopsies may only sample suspicious tissue, while in others, the entire area of abnormal tissue may be removed during the procedure.

Often, X rays, ultrasound, or other diagnostic techniques commonly in use by gastroenterologists and other physicians disclose growths or other suspicious findings that should be sampled by biopsy for further analysis. In most cases, though not all, the doctor is able to take a sample during endoscopy.

With the endoscope in the precise location of the tissue to be sampled, a biopsy forceps or special brush is put down an internal channel in the endoscope. The doctor then cuts or scrapes away a suitable sample of the tissue and withdraws it through the channel.

In many cases, small growths or suspicious-looking areas not apparent in X rays or other diagnostic techniques are first discovered during endoscopic examination of the upper digestive tract. In these situations, tissue samples are immediately taken and the patient spared the cost and discomfort of a separate procedure. Fortunately, most (though not all) tissues that the gastroenterologist might wish to biopsy are accessible by the endoscopic method.

Usually the endoscopic procedure takes less than a half hour. At its conclusion, the endoscope is withdrawn and you are allowed to relax while the effects of the medication and sedatives begin to wear off. During this time, you should not eat or drink anything. Similarly, since the effects of sedation may not have worn off completely by the time you are able to leave, it is probably prudent to go home by taxi or arrange to have someone meet you at the doctor's office.

With the possible exception of mild hoarseness or sore throat that may last a day or two, most remaining effects, if any, are usually mild and brief.

Through training and extensive experience, the physician knows the appearance of a normal, healthy digestive tract, as well as of any abnormalities which may have been observed. Results of fiber-optic endoscopy are therefore commonly discussed with the patient following the test.

The results of any biopsy samples taken are determined by a medical specialist called a pathologist. Using specialized techniques, the pathologist prepares the samples, then examines them microscopically and characterizes the tissue as to type and whether it is cancerous (malignant) or noncancerous (benign). The pathologist is also able to detect any inflammation or infection that may be present in the tissue. These results are then provided to the gastroenterologist. Several days may be required, however, for results of laboratory analysis of tissue samples to be known. When performed by a properly trained and experienced pathologist, the information obtained from a tissue sample taken by biopsy is highly accurate.

Fiber-optic endoscopy is not without risk of complications. You may be advised to watch carefully for any indication of bleeding for several days if biopsies have been taken. Such indications would include black, tarry stools or bloody vomit. Other rare complications include perforation and infection.

Ultrasound (Sonogram)

Ultrasound is a relatively recent though well-established diagnostic technique widely used alone or in conjunction with other tests.

Sonography ("sound-writing") uses essentially the same technology developed to locate and track submarines. The basic principles are simple: a "beam" of sound (in this case, very high frequency sound that is inaudible to people) is directed into the abdomen from the skin surface of the body, strikes the internal organs and other structures, and bounces back in the direction from which it came. The same hand-held device (called a "transducer") which directs the beam is also equipped with a sensitive microphone to detect the returning "echoes." The information contained in these echoes is then fed through a computer to either a video monitor or pen recorder (similar to the devices that record earthquakes). What results is a "picture," which, when interpreted by an expert, contains a great deal of useful information regarding the condition of the internal organs.

Ultrasound uses no X rays and therefore avoids the risks associated with radiation. In fact, sonography is known to most people as the technique by which physicians are able to view unborn infants (a group particularly vulnerable to the dangers of radiation from X rays). No known risks to the patient are associated with ultrasound tests.

In its application to diagnosis of gastrointestinal problems, sonography is particularly helpful in showing the glands associated with digestion, including the gallbladder, pancreas, and liver.

As with other diagnostic tests of the gastrointestinal system, best results from the sonogram are obtained when the digestive tract is empty of all food at the time of the test. In preparation, the sonographer (or your doctor) will ask you to refrain from all food and drinks after the evening meal on the day before the test is scheduled. In addition, if the test is being done on the gall-bladder or pancreas, you'll be asked to make sure that the meal is fat-free.

Just before the test is to begin, you will be asked to recline on the examining table, and the sonographer (or assistant) will apply a clear, water-soluble gel to the abdomen. This substance eliminates the air at the skin's surface (air can distort the sound) and improves the conduction of the sound.

The sonographer holds the transducer and passes it back and forth lightly on the skin over the area to be examined. During the test, you will be asked to hold your breath while each "picture" is taken. In all likelihood, you will also be asked to change position so that different views of the organ being examined can be obtained.

As part of an ultrasound examination of the gallbladder, the doctor may administer a drug to make the organ contract as it would during the process of digestion. As with any prescribed drug, make sure your physician (and the sonographer, if they are not the same person) is aware of any allergies you may have. Some individuals may experience minor side effects from the drug (such as nausea or abdominal cramps).

The results of the test are determined by visual inspection of the video monitor or the graphic recordings. Through training and extensive experience, the physician knows the appearance of normal, healthy digestive glands as well as those affected by problems. On the basis of careful examination by an expert, ultrasound can help establish, for example, whether organs are of normal size; whether the ducts by which their secretions enter the digestive system are free of obstructions; and whether they are tumorous, inflamed, or infected.

Computed Tomographic Scanning
(CAT Scanning, CT Scanning)

CAT scanning is a recently developed technique that combines X rays with sophisticated computer analysis. A CAT scan is essentially many X rays taken of the body from many directions.

The information from all these X rays is then analyzed by a computer, and a complete and very detailed picture of the internal organs is synthesized, shown on a video screen, and printed onto an X-ray plate.

CAT scanning uses X rays; therefore, as with all X-ray procedures, there are risks, especially to young children and pregnant mothers.

In its application to upper gastrointestinal problems, CAT scanning is particularly helpful in showing glands associated with digestion, including the pancreas, liver, and gallbladder. As with other tests of the gastrointestinal system, the best results are obtained when the digestive tract is empty of all food at the time of the test. You will therefore be asked to refrain from eating and drinking after the evening meal on the day before the test is scheduled; you may be asked to drink some contrast material with that evening meal.

Just before the test is about to begin, you will be asked to recline on the examining table, and you may receive further contrast material through an intravenous line inserted into your arm. Do make sure your physician and others know of any allergies you may have.

During the procedure you will be surrounded by a large "donut"-shaped piece of equipment that will move, taking X rays at various sites along your body in order to build up a complete picture of the internal organs. The results of the test are determined by visual inspection of the video monitor and the X-ray plates. Through training and experience, the physician knows the appearance on CAT scans of the normal, healthy digestive glands; therefore, he may well be able to tell whether ducts of the digestive system are free of obstruction or whether organs are tumorous or inflamed.

Blood Test for Gastrin

Gastrin is a hormone (a specialized chemical messenger) that is secreted by the stomach in response to the entry of food. It is produced in one part of the stomach, circulated throughout the body in the bloodstream, and returned to the acid-producing part of the stomach, where it stimulates production and release of hydrochloric acid. The presence of sufficient stomach acid, in turn, serves to inhibit further release of gastrin. Through this system of checks and balances, concentrations of both gastrin and stomach acid are prevented from rising above what is required for the digestive process.

If you develop multiple or recurrent ulcers, your doctor may suggest the test to determine if you have Zollinger–Ellison syndrome, a rare disorder due to a gastrin-secreting tumor (see pages 33–35). In this case, your blood will have a high concentration of gastrin that would make the appearance of such ulcers a predictable outcome.

However, if your system produces no acid, as occurs in atrophic gastritis (see pages 35–36), you may also have high gastrin concentrations.

In preparation for the test, the doctor will ask that you refrain from all solids after the evening meal on the day before the test is scheduled.

The test involves drawing a small sample of blood from a vein, usually in the arm. The concentration of gastrin in the sample is determined by a laboratory. Since the range of gastrin concentration normally expected to be present in blood is well established, test results are obtained by comparison of the sample of the accepted standard. Individuals with Zollinger–Ellison syndrome and atrophic gastritis may have gastrin levels that are up to several hundred times higher than normal.

Endoscopic Retrograde Cholangiography and Pancreatography (ERCP)

ERCP is a way of examining the bile and pancreatic ducts without surgery. It is a diagnostic procedure used when other tests raise suspicions that a blockage has occurred in the ducts draining the liver, gallbladder, or pancreas. Such blockages commonly occur as a result of gallstones, tumors, and a variety of other causes. In some cases, these blockages may be relieved by use of specialized tools passed through the endoscope and thus save the patient an operation.

This test requires the combined use of fiber-optic endoscopy (see pages 66–70) and X-ray studies, neither of which alone is able to provide the desired diagnostic information.

The fiber-optic endoscope, a thin, flexible viewing system contained in a tube less than a half-inch thick, is introduced into the patient's digestive tract through the mouth. Under the guidance of the gastroenterologist, it is advanced down the esophagus, through the stomach, and into the duodenum, where the common outlet for the bile duct and pancreatic gland is located. While watching the process through the endoscope, the doctor threads a narrow catheter (solid tube) into the opening of the duct and injects a contrast agent (see page 77). Without the contrast agent, the soft tissues of the duct would not be visible.

X-ray studies of the bile duct, pancreatic duct, or both (as appropriate) are then made, and any abnormalities will then be visible on the X-ray "picture."

Because it utilizes X rays, there is some slight risk associated with the ERCP test. X rays are a form of radiation that causes some degree of damage to the body; the greater the exposure, the greater the damage. Moreover, damage from X rays is cumulative over a period of years and poses particular danger to pregnant women, nursing mothers, and others.

Similarly, fiber-optic endoscopy is not without risk. If the duct from the pancreas is blocked, introduction of the contrast medium may cause acute pancreatitis (see pages 46–49). Similarly, if the bile duct is completely blocked, infection may occur. Other complications may include unexpected bleeding following endoscopic papillotomy (removal of gallstones without surgery) and perforation of the digestive tract, among others. To minimize these risks, ERCP should be performed only by a properly licensed, board-certified (or board-eligible) gastroenterologist.

In most cases, the combined procedures require less than an hour to complete. After the tests, you will be allowed to relax while the effects of the medication and sedatives used during endoscopy begin to wear off. You should not eat or drink during this period. Because the effects of the medication may not have worn off completely by the time you are able to leave, it is probably prudent to go home by taxi or have someone meet you at the doctor's office. With the possible exception of mild hoarseness or sore throat that may last a day or two, most remaining effects, if any, are usually mild and short-lived.

Vitamin B-12 Absorption Test (Schilling Test)

This test is used for individuals suffering from pernicious anemia, a condition due to vitamin B-12 deficiency. This deficiency can be due to lack of a particular stomach secretion (intrinsic factor), which must combine with B-12 before the vitamin can be absorbed later in the digestive process by the small intestine.

In preparation for the test, you will be required to abstain from food for the preceding twelve hours. You will be given an oral dose of vitamin B-12 that has been "tagged" with a small amount of radiation. After an hour or two, the doctor will administer a second dose of vitamin B-12, this one by injection into the muscle. You will be instructed to collect all urine for the next twenty-four hours, which will be used for laboratory analysis.

Test results are determined by the amount of "tagged" vitamin B-12 found in the urine. If less than 2 percent has been absorbed by the body during digestion, an absorption problem exists, but it may not be due to lack of intrinsic factor.

To test whether lack of intrinsic factor is the underlying cause of the poor absorption, the test is repeated. Everything is done as in the earlier test except that intrinsic factor is added to the oral dose. If the quantities of "tagged" vitamin B-12 appearing in the urine are now above 8 percent, lack of intrinsic factor is proved to be the underlying cause.

The small amount of radioactivity used in this test poses no known health risk. In a matter of a day or less, all traces of radioactivity have been eliminated from the body.

Tests of Esophageal Sensitivity and Acid Reflux

Tests of acid reflux are done to determine if a patient's symptoms are due to esophagitis and, if so, whether this condition is due to backflow (reflux) and retention in the esophagus of digestive juices from the stomach.

Definitive diagnosis may require combined information obtained through the use of several different tests.

BERNSTEIN TEST: The Bernstein test is used to determine whether the patient's esophagus is abnormally sensitive to stomach acid. A dilute solution of hydrochloric acid (similar to the acid normally in the stomach) is introduced into the esophagus through a tube. If the patient reports pain, esophagitis or a related condition (such as esophageal ulcer) is identified as the cause of the patient's symptoms.

MANOMETRY: This test measures pressure within the esophagus, allows the physicians to record the muscular contractions by which food and liquid are moved down the gullet during swallowing, and measures the constriction and relaxation of the lower esophageal sphincter.

A finding of weak muscular action by the esophagus in moving food through the gullet into the stomach, particularly in combination with inappropriate patterns of constriction and relaxation of the sphincter, strengthens suspicions that these factors are involved in the patient's esophagitis.

ESOPHAGEAL pH MONITORING: As the name suggests, acidity (of which pH is a measure) in the esophagus is monitored.

A measured dose of acid similar to that produced by the body is infused into the stomach by means of a tube. A small electronic sensor able to detect and measure pH in the esophagus is passed down the gullet into position near the lower esophageal sphincter. If acid refluxes into the esophagus, the pH will fall. In another form of the test, the sensor is left in the esophagus for 24 hours and measurements made periodically throughout the day and night as the patient goes about all normal activities.

Backflow of acidic materials from the stomach into the esophagus is normal in all people. However, these materials quickly return to the stomach and, consequently, cause no problems. However, sustained high levels of acidity recorded by the sensor indicate that refluxed material is being retained in the esophagus and is the likely cause of the esophagitis.

Percutaneous Transhepatic Cholangiogram

This test is a method your doctor can use to determine whether jaundice (yellowing of the skin and eyes) is due to a disease of the liver or to a blocked bile duct.

This test utilizes X rays to help the physician locate the ducts of the liver and to determine whether they are clear or obstructed. It is performed in the hospital.

Before the test begins, you will be administered a sedative. You are then placed on your back on the X-ray table and given an injection to numb the intervening skin, muscle, and capsule of the liver. Since it may be necessary to tilt the table during the procedure, you are secured to prevent slipping.

When the skin is numb, the doctor will ask you to exhale and hold very still while a needle is pushed through the tissue of the upper abdomen into the liver. The path of the needle is carefully guided by the doctor, who is able to observe its progress by means of a fluoroscope (a device that shows a continuous X ray). If a liver duct is located, a contrast agent is injected and one or more X rays taken. (The "contrast agent" is a substance that fills the hollow ducts and makes them stand out clearly on the X ray. Because this test makes use of such a substance, it is one of a group of such tests called "X-ray contrast studies.") If the duct is unobstructed, the contast agent will flow through the liver down the bile passageway into the duodenum.

Most patients experience very little, if any, discomfort during the procedure except for the needle-jab to administer the anesthetic. However, it will be necessary for you to remain under observation in the hospital. For several hours, you will have to lie flat, since bleeding or leakage of bile or infection are possible, through uncommon, complications.

Oral Cholecystography

This test is used to assess the general functioning of the gall-bladder as well as the duct system by which it receives bile from the liver and delivers it to the duodenum. It is used when symptoms of biliary tract disease, such as gallbladder colic, develop.

An oral cholecystectogram involves the use of X rays to help the physician visualize the gallbladder and associated system of ducts. Since these structures are comprised of soft tissue, they will show up as only vague shapes and shadows on the X ray. To make these structures stand out clearly for careful visual examination by the physician, special substances called "contrast agents" are used.

For approximately twenty-four hours before the test, you will be required to limit your intake of fat. Then, following the evening meal on the day preceding the test, you will be asked to take a number of pills containing a special contrast agent. By the morning of the test, the contrast should be visible in the gallbladder when X rays are taken (if it is not visible, the test is repeated with a larger dose).

You are then given a meal, and X rays of the gallbladder are taken at quarter-hour intervals. During the test, you may be asked to change positions several times. Generally, the information required by the doctor can be obtained in less than an hour.

The results of the test are determined by visual inspection by the doctor of the X rays. Normally, the gallbladder will empty its contents into the duodenum in response to the meal. If a gallstone or other obstruction is present, it should be visible on the X ray.

Because it utilizes X rays, there is some slight risk associated with oral cholecystography. X rays are a form of radiation that causes some degree of damage to the body; the greater the exposure, the greater the damage. Moreover, damage from X rays is cumulative over a period of years and poses particular dangers to young children, adolescent girls whose breasts are developing, and pregnant women.

While the benefit of this test usually outweighs the risk, for your protection it is important to discuss with the doctor any and all previous exposure you have had to radiation, including earlier X rays. This simple step can help assure that risks are maintained at an acceptable level.

The use of ultrasound (see pages 70–71) is gradually reducing the need to perform oral cholecystography as a diagnostic test.

Red Cell Scan Test

This diagnostic test is a method for locating the source of bleeding that has eluded detection by other techniques. Even fiber-optic endoscopy (pages 66–70), which provides the doctor with a direct view of the interior of the digestive tract, may be ineffective in finding the source of intermittent bleeding, unless bleeding happens to occur during the examination.

The red cell scan test is one of a growing number of diagnostic tests that come from the field of nuclear medicine, a relatively new specialty of medicine in which radionuclides (or "radioactive tracers," as they are sometimes called) play a central role. These materials, which can be introduced into the body in a variety of ways, including injection into the blood, emit small amounts of radiation which can be detected by devices that are sensitive to their radioactive emissions. In this test, radioactive tracers are injected into the bloodstream to "label" the red blood cells. By monitoring the digestive system, the precise point at which the blood enters the tract can then be determined and further corrective action taken, as appropriate.

The small amount of radioactive material used in this test poses about the same degree of risk as that associated with X rays.

Medication

It is crucial that you tell your doctor not only what drugs you are allergic to, if any, but the names of all the drugs you are taking, especially if they were prescribed by another doctor. Some drugs can have life-threatening interactions with other drugs, so be sure your physician knows about any medication you are on. If you have any doubts as to what they are or have trouble remembering their names or dosages, bring them in for your doctor's inspection.

Don't forget to mention any over-the-counter preparations you are taking: antacids, constipation remedies, aspirin, mineral or vitamin supplements. Medicines can interact with each other, causing undesirable, even dangerous, effects.

If you are or become pregnant, you should discuss with your doctor the possible effects of all prescribed medicines. Since the developing fetus is particularly sensitive to the effects of drugs, all medications should be thoroughly reconsidered and the appropriate action taken with the advice of your doctor.

Be careful to follow the instructions you are given regarding dosage. Do not increase the number of tablets or capsules you take without your doctor's advice. When it comes to medicines, more is not necessarily better and, in fact, may be dangerous.

If you have ever had an allergic reaction to a drug, be sure to inform your doctor. In most cases, a more suitable drug of equal value for your care is available and can be prescribed instead.

In reading and discussing drugs, you must know the difference between generics and brand names. The generic is the name a drug is given at its first discovery or concoction in a laboratory. It identifies the drug's unique chemistry and distinguishes it from all others. When the generic is marketed, however, it is given another name, a brand name. In the descriptions of specific medications which follow, both the generic and a representative brand name are given in most cases.

When the Food and Drug Administration approves a drug for sale and use, generally one drug manufacturer has developed it and is licensed to sell it. The drug is then sold under a brand name but with its generic name cited on the package as well. A number of years after its release, however, a drug becomes public property and other manufacturers can sell it also. At that point, there are likely to be a number of brand names under which the drug is sold. To make matters even more complicated, some manufacturers may sell the drug under its generic name and not adorn it with a brand name. As a general rule, once the original patent has expired, generic drugs are less expensive than brand names.

In the following pages, drugs are grouped according to their major effect on the digestive tract. There is, for example, a category for drugs that inhibit acid secretion and another for those that are mucosal coating agents. The drugs listed are representative of those in the group but do not necessarily represent all such drugs.

Potential Side Effects

The potential side effects of the drugs used in treating disorders of the upper GI tract are extremely diverse. While a catalogue of the potential side effects of many drugs can be frightening, a little knowledge and understanding of them can go a long way toward alleviating much of the concern.

Your doctor is by far your best guide through the complicated subject of potential untoward side effects. He or she will discuss with you the major side effects of the medicine being prescribed for your treatment. Your doctor will sometimes also deal with less likely side effects simply because they are dangerous, albeit rare.

The potential side effects of many drugs are usually listed on the package insert or printed on the container. Read them carefully for complete information on all known side effects. Any unusual changes or discomforts should be reported to your physician immediately upon their appearance. The doctor may decide it is not necessary to change your drug, but when armed with complete knowledge of your condition, he or she is certainly in a better position to advise you.

Antacids (Acid Neutralizers)

Antacid drugs are those capable of neutralizing acid and are therefore useful in treating conditions involving high acidity (such as ulcers, gastritis, and esophagitis) by neutralizing the effects of acid. Most can be purchased over-the-counter—that is, without a doctor's prescription. They are among the most widely used drugs in America, and the familiarity which most people have with brand names and active ingredients of these products (to say nothing of jingles and animated characters) is a reminder of how aggressively they are marketed.

Among the many products in this group are Gelusil, Maalox, Mylanta, Riopan Plus, Camalox, Di-Gel, Amphojel, Titralac, Tums, and Rolaids.

A number of chemical compounds produce the desired result, although those using magnesium (for example, magnesium trisilicate), aluminum (aluminum hydroxide), or calcium are among the most common.

Although all three groups of compounds are effective in achieving the desired effect of neutralizing acid, each produces characteristic side effects that may worsen other symptoms of the disorder for which they are being taken. Magnesium compounds commonly cause diarrhea as a side effect and should not be used when this is already a problem. Such compounds may, however, be a good choice if constipation is a problem. Aluminum and calcium products, on the other hand, tend to produce constipation as a side effect and should not be taken when this condition is present. They may be a good choice, however, if diarrhea is a problem.

Many popular products combine the use of both aluminum or calcium and magnesium compounds to cancel out the undesirable side effects of each. In addition, many add the drug simethicone or similar agents to combat gas in the digestive tract.

Antacids come in tablet, liquid, and powder (to be mixed with water) form; the latter two types are the quickest to take effect. Antacids are taken between meals for symptomatic relief of hyperacidity or as recommended by your doctor. Since the potency (that is, how much acid a given quantity of the medicine can neutralize) varies widely, ask your doctor or pharmacist which preparation is best for you.

Antacids interfere with the absorption of many other kinds of drugs and should not be taken with certain medications. Consult your doctor or pharmacist with regard to the prescribed medications you may be taking. Similarly, some products may contain sodium and should not be used by those who are limiting their sodium (salt) intake.

Mucosal Coating Agents

The effect of drugs in this category is to provide a barrier between the lining of the gastrointestinal tract and the chemicals that ulcerate it or, alternately, to enhance the body's natural barrier.

SUCRALFATE
This drug coats and adheres to the ulcer base. Its effectiveness comes from a combination of several properties. It produces a physical barrier which makes it more difficult for acid to reach the lining of the digestive tract. It also reduces the damaging effects of the digestive enzyme pepsin, thereby lessening the challenge to the tract's natural defenses. Finally, it stimulates the production of prostaglandins (page 91).

Antispasmodic Drugs (Muscle Relaxants)

Antispasmodics are drugs that inhibit gastrointestinal motility (the muscular activity of the digestive tract that moves food along) or muscular activity of the digestive glands. These drugs are commonly prescribed for conditions in which spasm or contractions of the muscles cause, or contribute to, the problem. Such conditions include functional disorders.

Many of the prescribed drugs in this category are anticholinergics that block the action of acetylcholine, a substance essential for the transmission of nerve impulses. Since the muscles move in response to nerve commands, the effect of the anticholinergics is to block receipt of the information channel by which they are stimulated into action. The muscle, poised and capable, remains at rest. Clidinium bromide (Quarzan) is an example of one such drug.

Other types of antispasmodics, such as papaverine hydro-chloride, act directly on the muscle. Some of these drugs are derived from opium.

Antispasmodics are often combined with antacids, antiemetics (drugs which reduce vomiting) or other drugs.

Many of these drugs have side effects that should be avoided by particular individuals. Their use should be discussed with a doctor.

Acid-Inhibiting Drugs

H2 BLOCKERS

These drugs are used in the treatment of ulcers and other digestive disorders in which it is necessary to reduce the amount of acid produced or released by the stomach. Among the products in this group are cimetidine (Tagamet), ranitidine (Zantac), and famotidine (Pepsid).

The production and release of stomach acid is triggered by several hormones (chemical messengers), including histamine, a hormone produced in the stomach. In order for histamine to have the desired effect, it must first bind to a specific histamine receptor (a specialized sensor) on each of the cells. This receptor is called an H2 receptor. It is only after histamine has bound to the H2 receptor that the cell begins producing and releasing acid.

H2 blockers, as the name implies, block this activating mechanism by occupying the histamine (H2) receptor, so that histamine cannot bind to it. The cell, though poised and capable, remains at rest.

These drugs are extremely effective in reducing stomach acid secretion and in subsequent healing of peptic ulcers, although their beneficial effect is somewhat greater on duodenal ulcers than gastric ulcers.

Few, if any, side effects are experienced by most users and, as a result, they can be used in almost complete safety. When side effects do occur, they may include headaches, dizziness, confusion, or rash, and, rarely, other more serious effects. When large doses are administered to men, cimetidine tends to promote undesirable side effects, including the development of breasts and impotence. Once again, the greatest effectiveness of anticholinergics is with duodenal, rather than gastric, ulcers.

The introduction of H2 blockers in the late 1970s represented a major step in the treatment of ulcer and have all but replaced all other forms of drug therapy.

ANTICHOLINERGICS

These drugs, of which propantheline bromide is an example, inhibit acid secretion by blocking the action of acetylcholine, a substance essential for the transmission of nerve impulses.

Acetylcholine plays the same role in triggering the acid-making cells as histamine except, of course, a different, but functionally equivalent receptor is involved. The effect of the anticholinergics is to block receipt of the information channel by which the acid-producing cell is stimulated into action. In this case, as with histamine H2 receptor antagonists, the cell, poised and capable, remains at rest.

However, acetylcholine is less effective in stimulating acid production than histamine. Blocking its action results in a much smaller reduction of total acid output from the cells.

The use of anticholinergics has declined since the introduction of the H2 blockers, which have fewer side effects. Side effects of the anticholinergics include dry eyes and mouth, headache, nausea, vomiting, and rapid heartbeat.

METOCLOPRAMIDE

Metoclopramide is a drug that works by increasing lower esophageal pressure and speeding the passage of food out of the stomach. It has been shown to improve esophagitis.

Surgical Procedures

Gastric or duodenal ulcer, biliary tract disease, cancer, and other disorders of the digestive tract can have dangerous, painful, or disabling consequences. In some cases, surgery is the best or only course of effective treatment.

First of all, a preliminary determination must be made in conjunction with your doctor. Among the questions to be answered are: Will surgery help me? What are the benefits I can expect from surgery? Will I be cured? Have all the nonsurgical alternatives been explored, including medication and changes in diet and lifestyle? Does it make more sense to have the surgery later? If you and your doctor decide that surgery makes sense for you, he or she will refer you to a surgeon.

We all have some sort of natural fear of surgery, which can be greatly and unduly increased by worry. Modern surgery and anesthesia are very safe, though certainly not without risk. Thoroughly discuss all aspects of the operation with your doctor—the anesthetic to be used, the length of the recuperative period, and the degree of risk. By all means, gather all the information you need to make an informed decision.

Remember that while surgical procedures for ulcers and other problems of the upper GI tract have progressed greatly, miracles are still in the province of religion rather than medicine. While some problems may be helped significantly, it is not always possible to restore the system to 100 percent perfection or to prevent recurrence of the problem.

Detailed discussion of the surgical procedures used in the treatment of gastrointestinal problems is clearly beyond the scope of this book. It may be helpful, however, when confronting the possibility of surgery, to have some idea of the objectives of these surgical procedures and what they may involve.

Since the underlying cause of peptic ulcer is a relative overproduction of acid, surgical treatment of this condition is aimed at reducing the amount of acid. From a surgical point of view, this can be accomplished in one of two ways: either by blocking the nerve impulses from the brain which stimulate the stomach to produce acid; or by removing some, or all, of the acid-producing tissues of the stomach itself.

While thousands of operations are performed each year to treat ulcer, the variety of operations used is relatively small, with only two or three procedures accounting for more than 90 percent of the total. These procedures, and several notable variations, are described in the pages that follow.

Vagotomy

The vagus (from the Latin, meaning "wandering") nerve plays two important functions with regard to the stomach: it stimulates secretion of acid; and it controls the muscular action by which the stomach is able to empty itself into the duodenum.

Vagotomy is a surgical procedure in which the vagus nerve is severed. Severing the nerve greatly reduces the production of acid.

However, because vagotomy also affects the ability of the stomach to empty its contents normally, the surgeon must provide for this function. One commonly used technique for ensuring proper drainage involves enlarging the stomach's natural outlet (pylorus) so that semidigested food passes easily into the duodenum. This combined procedure is called a truncal vagotomy (since the entire "trunk" of the nerve has been severed) and pyloroplasty.

Two variations of this basic surgical procedure are coming into more widespread use. One of these, called selective vagotomy, involves severing only the nerve fibers going to the stomach, thus leaving intact the fibers that serve other functions elsewhere. Although surgical enlargement of the stomach outlet is still required to ensure proper drainage, the advantage of this procedure is that other functions of the vagus nerve are unimpaired by the surgery.

The other variations of this procedure, called highly selective vagotomy (or parietal cell vagotomy), severs only those nerve fibers going to the acid-producing cells themselves. This procedure, though more delicate to perform, does not affect the normal muscular activity of the stomach; as a consequence, there is no need to enlarge the stomach outlet to ensure proper drainage.

Vagotomy, both with and without pyloroplasty, is a widely used and generally quite successful surgical treatment of gastric and duodenal ulcers. However, in up to 10 percent of the cases in which it is used, the ulcer may recur.

Gastrectomy

As mentioned previously, the second major approach to the surgical treatment of peptic ulcer is removal of some portion of the tissue of the stomach itself, thereby reducing the stomach's capacity to produce acid. In fact, until vagotomy came into widespread use, partial or total gastrectomy (stomach removal) was the most widely used surgical treatment. At present, the generally accepted procedure when a gastrectomy is performed is to also perform a vagotomy.

In gastrectomy, the connection between the stomach and the duodenum is severed, some portion of the lower stomach removed and the cut edges of the remaining portion reconnected to the duodenum so that proper drainage is maintained. In some cases in which the duodenum is badly ulcerated, the surgeon may bypass this area and reconnect the stomach at a point slightly further along the intestinal tract (the jejunum). If this procedure (called a gastrojejunostomy) is chosen, the severed end of the duodenum is simply sewn closed and left in place. Although it varies from case to case, from 40 percent to 70 percent of the stomach is generally removed in a partial gastrectomy. Since the lower portion of stomach is called the antrum, partial gastrectomy may also be referred to as an antrectomy.

Gastrectomy is a highly effective surgical treatment for ulcer. However, because it involves more extensive surgery than vagotomy, it carries a somewhat higher risk. In addition, gastrectomy often produces an unpleasant side effect called the "dumping syndrome." The symptoms of the syndrome are quite pronounced: shortly after eating, patients who have undergone gastrectomy may feel faint, even to the point of having to lie down. This early effect is probably related to rapid fluid changes in the body. Later, the person may experience discomfort as the food consumed at the meal flows into the intestine.

Gastric Bypass Surgery

Gastric bypass is a surgical procedure in which a detour is created to bypass the outlet of the stomach. It may be done, for example, when an inoperable tumor interferes with, or blocks completely, the passage of food into the intestine. It is not a form of treatment for the underlying problem (the tumor, in this case) but rather a method for ameliorating some of its symptoms.

When the gastric bypass procedure is performed, the remaining portion of the stomach is generally connected to a new opening created by the surgeon somewhat further along the intestinal tract beyond the duodenum (the procedure is called gastro-jejunostomy).

Cholecystectomy

Cholecystectomy is the surgical removal of the gallbladder. It is often recommended as the preferred course of treatment for patients who develop cholecystitis and other serious complications of gallbladder disease.

Generally, the patient is admitted to the hospital and an evaluation made of whether or not emergency surgery is required. If it is not, painkillers are administered to provide symptomatic relief, and the person is treated to reduce the inflammation and any infection that may be present. Since cholecystitis is likely to recur, the person will be urged to schedule the surgery at a convenient time in the near future.

Cholecystectomy is done through an incision in the center or upper right part of the abdomen. After the gallbladder has been exposed and its duct tied off and severed, it is removed. During the operation, which usually takes about one and a half hours, the surgeon will order X-ray studies of the ducts. If stones are found, the surgeon will open the common bile duct from the liver and remove them.

A small percentage of patients who have their gallbladder surgically removed experience so-called "postcholecystectomy syndrome." For reasons poorly understood, these individuals have the same or similiar symptoms as before the removal of the gallbladder.

Esophageal Surgery

A tube may be inserted into the esophagus when a stricture due to an inoperable tumor threatens to close the esophagus.

Another surgical procedure done to eliminate serious acid reflux into the esophagus from the stomach is called fundoplication, in which the top of the stomach (the fundus) is folded in such a way that acid can no longer enter the esophagus.

What the Future May Hold

The Causes of Ulcer

Many of those who are involved in clinical care or research on gastrointestinal disorders have long had suspicions that bacteria are somehow involved in the development of gastric ulcer. While provocative findings occasionally fuel new speculations, conclusive proof continues to elude researchers.

In one recent study, for example, a variety of bacteria often found in the digestive system of sufferers of gastric ulcer was given to two healthy volunteers. Both developed gastritis, an inflammation of the acid-producing portion of the stomach.

The theory that has won support thus far holds that when these bacteria enter the stomach wall, they cause generalized chronic gastritis in some susceptible people.

Some physicians believe such bacteria may also cause ulcers, but others remain skeptical. Much research is being conducted into this area at the moment.

Treatment of Ulcers

OMEPRAZOLE: This is a new and potent acid-inhibiting drug currently undergoing tests to determine its suitability for widespread use. Omeprazole is up to ten times more effective in suppressing acid production than H2 blockers, which themselves represented a quantum leap in ulcer care when they were introduced some years ago.

The chemical action of omeprazole is on a particular enzyme (hydrogen potassium ATPase) responsible for the final step in the release of hydrogen ions (electrically charged atoms of hydrogen). By blocking this final step in acid production, the drug effectively blocks gastric acid secretion.

Although only preliminary data are available, omeprazole seems to be effective in treating even such extreme conditions of overproduction of acid as those associated with Zollinger–Ellison syndrome (see pages 33–35).

PROSTAGLANDINS: Prostaglandins are substances produced by the stomach (and by other parts of the body). They have a dual capacity of decreasing secretion of acid and, at the same time, of stimulating the production of mucus and other neutralizing secretions that provide natural protection against the acid's damaging properties.

The use of prostaglandins to promote and accelerate healing of areas in the digestive tract damaged by gastric ulcer is relatively new but, as more becomes known through medical research, it may prove to be another important advance in the care of these problems.

More research will be needed before the future role of these drugs in ulcer care is clear.

Finding the "Ideal" Approach to Treatment of Ulcer

Today there are basically three schools of thought regarding how treatment of ulcer should be approached. Some believe that acid secretion should be strongly suppressed for a prolonged period. This group subscribes to the "no acid, no ulcer" school of thought.

The laboratory research done on potent acid suppressors such as H2 blockers and omeprazole raise concern that aggressive acid suppression may give rise to conditions in which certain types of bacteria flourish in the GI tract, and that the products produced by these bacteria may be related to the development of cancer.

A second school of thought favors more moderate suppression of acid production, principally during the eight- to twelve-hour period during the night when acid production in the person with duodenal ulcer is often high and there is no food in the system to act as a neutralizer. At night, when the person is at rest, a smaller dose of medication gives results that could only be achieved during the day by giving a larger dose.

Finally, there are those who favor the use of drugs such as sucralfate (page 83) that do not have a direct effect on acid secretion.

Although suppression of acid production has been the primary method for treating gastric ulcer in the past, it is likely that in the future a more balanced approach will emerge in which acid suppression is balanced with healing and maintaining the health of the lining of the GI tract.

Treatment of Gallstones

Continued development of safe and effective oral drugs to dissolve gallstones undoubtedly will reduce the considerable number of people who must currently undergo surgery for this reason. Research is continuing on two such drugs, chenodeoxycholic acid and ursodeoxycholic acid (pages 54–55), which are chemically similar to bile acids made in the liver. These bile acids normally serve to keep cholesterol from precipitating out of the bile solution and forming a "stone."

Diagnosis of GI Disorders

There is no question that advances in technology in such fields as nuclear medicine, computer-aided analysis, microminiaturization (drastic size reduction of diagnostic and research tools allowing them, for example, to be swallowed), and video will contribute to the ease and accuracy of diagnosing gastrointestinal disorders.

CHAPTER 3

Other Resources

Digestive disorders account for the largest amount of time lost from work and are the cause of nearly one of every five hospital admissions. Not reflected in these facts, of course, are the millions who suffer in silence or whose digestive disorders progress without frank symptoms.

The fact is that because so many are afflicted there is a vast literature and a vast array of drugs and other products to meet the needs of sufferers. In addition, a diversity of healthcare professionals and associations have evolved to help the millions of people with ulcers or some other form of gastrointestinal disorder. It is these individuals and organizations that are the focus of this chapter.

This chapter is divided into two sections. The first concerns the professionals, those individuals who play specific roles in your healthcare, from the familiar family doctor and the nurse to such specialists as the gastroenterologist, the radiologist, and the discharge planner. It is in this section that you will meet the professionals who are, in essence, the guides who will help you negotiate the tricky medical landscape.

The second section introduces the organizations out there that may be of help to you. Some of them, like the American Digestive Disease Society or the Center for Ulcer Research and Education, exist solely to advance the interests of individuals suffering from gastrointestinal problems of one sort or another. Some of these associations offer support groups, most have newsletters or other publications, many sponsor research, and virtually all can offer you some valuable services in getting the best care possible.

As someone dealing with a gastrointestinal disorder, you may have to deal with a series of events that unfold, each with its own surprises. In this chapter you will get a broader picture of the services available to you and the kinds of specific help available from medical professionals or from national or local organizations.

The Professionals

We live in a world where specialization rules. While the notion of a "family doctor" has made a notable comeback in recent years, the prevailing wisdom still argues strongly for expert consultation, especially when your complaint is unusual or serious.

If your condition is a "garden-variety" gastric ulcer in which, say, antacids and some degree of care in avoiding foods that disagree with you are all that is needed to relieve your symptoms and allow the ulcer to heal, your family doctor is probably quite able to provide you with the medical advice and care you need. (These days, by the way, the family doctor is often termed the "primary care physician".) However, if your digestive disorder requires specialized methods of diagnosis or treatment, your doctor undoubtedly will refer you to one or more specialists.

Today, there are over forty different medical specialties and subspecialties that, as organized groups, set the rules for specialized training and examinations that must be met by incoming younger doctors before they are certified as specialists in their own rights. Among the specialists that you, as a patient with a gastorintestinal disorder, may work with are a gastroenterologist, pathologist, and radiologist.

Each has a different period of required training and different types of examinations; the requirements are, of course, tailored to the nature of the discipline and are meant to ensure that those certified are competent. With pride in their discipline and with the desire to foster only the best possible performance, the various certifying bodies or boards often require years of practice under supervision and set very difficult examinations. In fact, "board certification" implies skills and knowledge that are, as a rule, above the level required for state licensing as a physician.

Another modern trend has been toward more and more specialization, even in the face of public demand for more generalists and family doctors. However, many older physicians, despite having devoted much of their professional life to certain fields of human illness, are not necessarily board certified; they may share or perhaps surpass the expertise of the younger, certified doctor. Thus, while it is well to be aware of your doctor's certificates and listings in specialty directories, such factors do not tell the whole story.

Gastroenterologist

The gastroenterologist is a specialist in internal medicine (an "internist") who has gone on to become a specialist in the diagnosis and treatment of diseases of the digestive system, including the esophagus, stomach, small and large intestines, liver, and pancreas. He or she not only has an M.D. degree but has also completed additional training in this specialty.

Becoming an internist involves spending a minimum of three years after medical school getting accredited training in the broad field of internal medicine. The three-year period is often divided into one year of internship and two of residency, but in any case the thirty-six months of training will have included at least twenty-four months of "meaningful patient responsibility." Two examinations must also be passed.

Having earned the right to be called an internist, the doctor who wishes to become a specialist in gastroenterology must complete two additional years of full-time graduate training in his field. There is another written test to be passed, and the candidate must have clinical competence attested to by the director of the gastroenterology program he or she attends. The result is a high level of expertise in the gastrointestinal diseases.

If you have any difficulty finding a qualified gastroenterologist, check with your county medical society or a local accredited hospital. If you are a member, the American Digestive Diseases Society can also help.

Often a gastroenterologist will work with a nurse who has

received special training in gastroenterology. In some cases, two or more gastroenterologists will pool their resources to work in a single office or clinic where X-ray resources, pathologists, and other healthcare providers with specialized skills vis-à-vis gastroenterology can be gathered together.

General Surgeon

Surgery deals with the treatment of injuries, disease, or malfunctions by means of surgical procedures. Surgery is used to preserve or restore lost function and to cure disease or malformations. The surgeon is a doctor who has undertaken substantial training following completion of the study of general medicine.

Anesthesiologist

The anesthesiologist is the medical specialist who administers the local or general anesthesia before and during the surgical procedure. Anesthesia serves to protect the patient from sensations of pain during the surgery and to relax the patient's body so that the surgeon can perform the operation. During the period that the patient is unconscious, the anesthesiologist monitors, manages, and supports the life functions. The anesthesiologist, like most physicians, is also trained to perform both cardiac and respiratory resuscitation in the event that it is required by the patient.

Pathologist

The pathologist is the medical specialist who examines body cells, tissues, and other body products to assess the degree to which disease has altered them. The pathologist uses specialized techniques to prepare samples provided by the gastroenterologist or surgeon, then subjects them to examination by microscope or other techniques. The information provided by the pathologist is often of major importance in determining the course of treatment for the patient.

Radiologist

The radiologist is a physician whose training and experience has prepared him or her to use X rays and other forms of radiant energy in the diagnosis and treatment of disease. This specialty is in the process of rapid change as a result of technological advances. The CAT scan, magnetic resonance imaging, ultrasound, scintillation scans, and other new techniques have made the radiologist one of the most important members of the health team.

Other Healthcare Professionals

There are a multitude of other healthcare providers whom you may meet in your travels across the medical landscape. If you are hospitalized and should require any special services as the release date approaches, you are likely to make the acquaintance of a *discharge planner*. The discharge planner is responsible for coordinating the services you will require for the transition from hospital environment to home. This responsibility runs the gamut from helping you fill out forms, to arranging for necessary equipment, to helping you cope with complex financial or family circumstances. Although the job designation is a fairly new one, social workers or nurses have long handled such responsibilities, and continue to do so.

In some cases, serious problems in our lives may indirectly affect our health. When the stress of chronic problems builds over time, it may affect health adversely by aggravating an existing problem, such as a tendency toward high blood pressure, or a stress-related ulcer. In cases of gastrointestinal problems where depression or other mental health concerns arise, a *medical social worker* may be called in. In some cases where the problem is more severe, a *psychologist* or *psychiatrist* may be consulted (the psychologist has a Ph.D.; the psychiatrist is an M.D. with a specialty in psychiatry).

No doubt a *pharmacist* will fill your prescriptions for drugs, and he or she can be a valuable source of information regarding the medication if there are things you don't understand.

The
Organizations

Make that call, write that letter, follow up on that lead, or telephone any of the following organizations if their concerns are yours. That is especially true if they are in your area.

While the attempt in this chapter is to cite the useful services these organizations offer you, space limitations do not allow for including everything. Once you have contacted one or more of these organizations, you may discover that they are sources, directly or indirectly, of a variety of kinds of help. They may offer you access to support groups, lectures, and any number of services or assistance.

Check your yellow pages, too, for local organizations. Ask your doctor and other patients for other sources.

There are many people like you out there. It is important that you not feel isolated: get to know your peers; they will understand you. And get all the help you can.

AMERICAN CANCER SOCIETY
777 3rd Avenue
New York, New York 10017
(800) 227-2345

The American Cancer Society is a national voluntary health association with local affiliates in every state. The society is involved in a variety of activities, among which are the publication and distribution of educational materials and educational programs directed to the prevention of cancer.

For information on materials, educational programs, and other services available through the society, call the local affiliate listed in your phone directory.

AMERICAN DIABETES ASSOCIATION, INC.
National Service Center
1660 Duke Street
Alexandria, Virginia 22314
(800) 232-3472

The American Diabetes Association (ADA) is a national voluntary health organization whose programs seek to improve the well-being of people with diabetes and their families. It is a not-for-profit association with affiliates in virtually every state.

Check your local telephone directory for the address of the ADA affiliate in your area. The affiliate can provide you with a variety of useful publications at little or no charge.

AMERICAN DIETETIC ASSOCIATION
430 North Michigan Avenue
Chicago, Illinois 60610
(312) 751-6166

The American Dietetic Association is a membership group of nutritionists and dietitians.

The association produces material and conducts educational programs designed to help people with special meal patterns or diet requirements specific to their needs. The organization can provide referral to local services and specialists in your area.

Write to the association for materials on proper nutrition and other subjects suitable for people with gastrointestinal disorders.

AMERICAN DIGESTIVE DISEASE SOCIETY
7720 Wisconsin Avenue
Bethesda, Maryland 20814
(301) 652-9293

The ADDS disseminates information about specific digestive disorders, including dietary recommendations and a program for stress and symptom management. It provides physician/specialist referrals and personal counseling to ADDS members and sponsors GUT-LINE, a telephone call-in information service for the public. It also publishes "Person to Person" brochures and six dietary plans.

AMERICAN HEART ASSOCIATION, INC.
7320 Greenville Avenue
Dallas, Texas 75231
(214) 750-5300

Local Heart Associations operate in every state. The associations support research on heart attack, stroke, and vascular disease, and offer a variety of educational materials including pamphlets and books. They also conduct community programs and public education in these and a variety of related subject areas with the objective of reducing health problems and disability from heart and blood vessel diseases.

If you wish to give up smoking, a known risk factor in many gastrointestinal disorders, the association can provide helpful pamphlets and other aids. Write or call your local Heart Association for more information.

AMERICAN MEDICAL ASSOCIATION
535 North Dearborn Street
Chicago, Illinois 60610
(312) 751-6000

In addition to producing and distributing educational materials to the public, the AMA, which is a membership organization of physicians, also serves as a source of information regarding specialists, facilities, and other matters relating to medicine.

Write to the AMA for information on gastrointestinal diseases or related medical matters, or if you need help in locating a physician or specialist in your area.

AMERICAN PHARMACEUTICAL ASSOCIATION
2215 Constitution Avenue, N.W.
Washington, D.C. 20037
(202) 628-4410

The association produces and distributes materials on a variety of drugs and related subjects. Write to the organization for information on brand name and generic drugs, over-the-counter preparations, drug interactions, child safety, or other matters relating to the use and abuse of medicines.

CENTER FOR ULCER RESEARCH AND EDUCATION (CURE) FOUNDATION
11661 San Vincente Boulevard, Suite 304
Los Angeles, California 90049
(213) 825-5091

The CURE Foundation supports research into the cause, cure, and prevention of peptic ulcer disease; sponsors conferences and symposia; and publishes educational materials, including an information brochure, "Are You an 'Ulcer' Person?"

DIGESTIVE DISEASE NATIONAL COALITION
c/o Slack, Inc.
1825 I Street, N.W.
Washington, D.C. 20006

The Digestive Disease National Coalition represents a variety of voluntary and professional disease organizations. It monitors relevant state and federal legislation, informs its members of important issues and events, and distributes information about digestive diseases to the public. The organization publishes a member newsletter and informational pamphlet.

GASTRO-INTESTINAL RESEARCH FOUNDATION
6 North Michigan Avenue, Suite 1318
Chicago, Illinois 60602
(312) 332-1350

The foundation supports research and training programs at the University of Chicago Medical Center, Section of Gastroenterology. It also sponsors educational activities for the public, and publishes a newsletter and a patient education pamphlet.

MEDIC-ALERT FOUNDATION
2323 Colorado Avenue
Turlock, California 95381-1009
(209) 668-3333

Medic-Alert is a nonprofit foundation that, for a (tax-deductible) fee, issues a Medic-Alert emblem which can be worn as a bracelet or necklace. The emblem bears the internationally recognized symbol of the medical profession on one side. Engraved on the reverse side, your medical condition, identification number, and a twenty-four-hour collect phone number are given. This phone number ensures that in the event of an emergency in which you are unable to speak, your medical records and the names of physicians and relatives to be contacted are instantly accessible to emergency and healthcare personnel treating you. Write to the foundation for further information.

NATIONAL CANCER INSTITUTE
Office of Cancer Communications
Building 31, Room 10A-18
9000 Rockville Pike
Bethesda, Maryland 20892
(800) 422-6237

Among its many activities, the National Cancer Institute publishes educational materials relating to the causes, diagnosis, treatment, and prevention of cancer, including cancer of the digestive system. Write or call the institute for a list of publications available free or at low cost.

NATIONAL COUNCIL ON ALCOHOLISM
12 West 21st Street
New York, New York 10010
(212) 206-6770

Among the objectives of the National Council on Alcoholism is the production and distribution of educational materials and programs designed to acquaint the public with the dangers of alcoholism and its consequences on health. Write to the council for a full listing of materials available free or at low cost.

NATIONAL DIGESTIVE DISEASES INFORMATION
  CLEARINGHOUSE
1255 23rd Street, N.W., Suite 275
Washington, D.C. 20037
(202) 296-1138

The National Digestive Diseases Information Clearinghouse is a service of the National Institute of Diabetes and Digestive and Kidney Diseases, National Institutes of Health. Mandated by Congress to coordinate a national effort to inform the public, patients and their families, and physicians and other healthcare providers, the clearinghouse works with other organizations to promote a wider understanding of digestive health and disease. The organization provides three major types of services: response to and referral of inquiries; development, review, and distribution of publications; and coordination of national resources.

Publications produced by the clearinghouse are carefully reviewed for scientific accuracy, appropriateness of content, and readability. Publications produced by sources other than the clearinghouse are also reviewed for scientific accuracy and are used, along with clearinghouse publications, to respond to information requests.

NATIONAL SELF-HELP CLEARINGHOUSE
33 West 42nd Street
New York, New York 10036
(212) 840-7606

The National Self-Help Clearinghouse is a referral center for all sorts of support groups. It can advise you of relevant professional organizations, community programs, and support groups operating in your area. It also publishes and distributes a directory. Write to the clearinghouse for further information.

NUTRITION INFORMATION SERVICE
234 Webb Building
University Station
Birmingham, Alabama 35294
(205) 934-3923

The Nutrition Information Service disseminates information about diet and nutrition to professionals, patients, and the public. It also conducts and participates in professional education activities.

OVEREATERS ANONYMOUS
4025 Spencer Street
Torrance, California 90503
(213) 542-8363

Set up along the lines of Alcoholics Anonymous, OA helps people to gain control of an aspect of their lives that can contribute to or worsen gastrointestinal disorders and jeopardize their general health. Much of the organization's work is done through support groups made up of people who share similar problems, concerns, failures, and successes.

CHAPTER 4

Self-Help

In a number of the digestive conditions discussed in Chapter 1, doctors do not yet know what triggers the development of the disorders. They are able to recognize the signs and symptoms of these health problems and treat them, but often they simply don't know why disease develops in one person rather than another.

In discussing each of these disorders, the known risk factors were identified. Often the risk factors include age, sex, family history, or race—factors about which we can do nothing. However, other risk factors, such as obesity, smoking, or excessive use of alcohol, can be brought under control or eliminated entirely. The success of one's own efforts in eliminating risk factors such as smoking or excessive alcohol consumption is often problematic; it is not easy to quit smoking or stop drinking. To help you in your efforts, you will find organizations and publications listed in Chapters 3 and 5 that provide you with additional information and assistance. Your doctor also may be able to offer guidance. Ultimately, though, it is up to you to confront these matters and get them under control.

The role of two additional factors in gastrointestinal disorders—psychological stress and diet—is somewhat less clear. There are those who are of the opinion that psychological stress is irrelevant to these illnesses, and others who hold the opinion that the relationship is clear, though scientifically unproven. Similarly, there are those who maintain that diet, too, is largely irrelevant, since there is no clear-cut evidence linking any particular diet or kind of food to the development of gastrointestinal disorders such as ulcer.

While further research is needed to determine the role of stress and diet in gastrointestinal illness, some helpful information is available.

Diet and Nutrition

The Balanced Diet

A proper, balanced diet makes anyone "healthier." Whether you are currently suffering from gastrointestinal problems or suffered from them in the past, you will be healthier (and probably happier, too) if you eat a sensible, varied diet that contains all the nutrients your body needs.

One of the easiest ways to assure you are eating a balanced diet is to eat, on a daily basis, the following foods:

- Two servings of protein (meat, fish, poultry, beans).
- Four to six servings of fruits or vegetables (at least one green leafy vegetable and one citrus fruit).
- Four to six servings of breads and cereals.
- Two servings of milk and dairy products (unless you are being treated for a disorder involving excess stomach acid, such as duodenal ulcer, in which case you should avoid milk).
- Six to eight glasses of water or other drinks.

Foods to Be Avoided or Minimized

There is no convincing evidence that diet causes gastrointestinal disorders, although, as we will see shortly, there are some foods or food constituents that appear to have a beneficial effect.

If you are under treatment for ulcer, avoid milk, high-protein foods, and beverages containing alcohol or caffeine (including colas) because they increase acid production. In addition, if you are under treatment for, or have a history of, digestive disorder, avoid or eliminate any food or beverage from your diet that seems to "disagree" with you.

Fiber

Much has been written about the health benefits of fiber. Classified as either water soluble or water insoluble, fiber (also called bulk or roughage) is found in abundance in a wide variety of foods, including dried beans (lentils, peas), vegetables (corn, winter squash, potato), whole grains, and many fruits and nuts. It is also found in unprocessed bran, whole wheat bread, prunes, and prune juice. The type of fiber that is insoluble in water (such as wheat bran) is not digested at all by the body but helps the digestive process and may reduce constipation.

Bran also may help prevent the formation of gallstones by reducing the cholesterol concentration of the bile. It is believed that as food releases cholesterol in the gastrointestinal tract, the indigestible fiber binds to the cholesterol. The fiber-bound cholesterol cannot be absorbed into the bloodstream and is simply carried through the intestine into the fecal matter and then excreted.

Another constituent in the diet that may be helpful in preventing formation of gallstones is lecithin. Lecithin, a substance rich in certain types of fats, helps to prevent cholesterol from precipitating out of the bile in the form of a gallstone.

Stress

What Is Stress?

Stress is a natural response that occurs in our bodies in reaction to life events and changing conditions. Conditions that can produce a stress reaction are called "stressors." Stressors may be either physical or psychological in nature. Common physical stressors include illness, injury, or infection; common psychological stressors include anxiety, fear, or depression.

Regardless of the source of stress, all stress produces essentially the same reaction, though in differing degrees. The stronger the stress (whether in real or perceived terms), the stronger the corresponding reaction it produces.

When we speak of stress in everyday conversation, we're generally referring to events or conditions that have a negative effect on us. However, happy events also trigger a response in our bodies. As far as our own body's reaction is concerned, a surprise birthday party or unexpected promotion can be just as stressful—though considerably more pleasant—than an argument at a traffic light.

What Does Stress Do to the Body?

A stress response is a series of physical changes that normally help mobilize us to adapt to changing conditions. Stress is essentially a defense mechanism that protects us by stimulating our nervous system to release certain hormones, or chemical messengers, which in turn act on the body to produce the extra energy needed to meet the new challenges presented by the stressors.

Everyone is familiar with the sensations of stress. Your head may pound and your forehead bead up with perspiration. But there are other reactions to stress that cannot be seen or felt quite so directly. These "hidden" reactions to stress include increased flow of blood in the lining of the digestive tract, increased digestive secretions, and, in some people, excessive acid secretion in the stomach.

These reactions may be easily handled by someone whose digestive system is sound; however, in an individual already suffering from an ulcer or another condition such as gastritis or duodenitis, each additional insult to injured or inflamed tissues is potentially the straw that breaks the camel's back.

Stress also has a psychological impact that causes some people to drink or smoke to excess, risk factors clearly associated with a number of GI problems.

While it cannot be said that stress bears a clear-cut cause-and-effect relationship to the development of ulcers or other gastrointestinal disorders, it seems reasonable to conclude that for some people, under some conditions, such a relationship does exist.

As someone troubled with gastrointestinal disorder, learning to combat the effects of stress is just one more aspect of your own self-help efforts.

Coping with Emotional Stress

Stress may be the result of life's highs and lows. Marriage, the birth of a baby, or the death of a parent are all emotionally stressful occurrences. Controlling stress and the impact it may have on your physical well-being is important.

There are some simple strategies that may help. At times they may be hard to follow, but try.

- Accept what you cannot change. No matter how willing you are to take on life's challenges, there's no point in doing battle with forces you cannot change. Accept the facts and use your energies to positive ends.
- Take life one day at a time. Try to focus on what is important today and not be distracted by the unknowns and uncertainties of next week or next year. In the same way, negotiate your way around the obstacles confronting you, taking each as it comes.
- Try to do something you enjoy each day. Life's little pleasures can sometimes make bigger problems seem less immense.
- Be reasonable in establishing goals and plans. Don't set goals that you can't possibly meet, as you'll only be disappointed when you fail and put pressure on yourself in the process.
- Incorporate a period of exercise into your daily schedule. Besides its beneficial effects on your general well-being, exercise can also help you to relax.

The ways in which one person deals with stress may not necessarily work for another. For some people, a quiet night at home with a good book is effective, while for others, an invigorating game of tennis seems to do the trick. As with the choice of foods in your diet, choose what works for you.

CHAPTER 5

Selected Print
and
Audiovisual Materials

If what you learned in the previous chapters of this book made you want to know more, there is an extensive library of print and audiovisual materials available to you.

The intent of this closing chapter is to provide you with specific sources for further information. The first section presents the available publications, ranging from pamphlets that require only minutes to read, to complex, full-length reference works. The concluding section lists audiovisual materials available in film, videocassette, or audiocassette format.

Both the print and audiovisual sections of this chapter are divided into subsections. The first subsection includes materials that offer information about various general aspects of the digestive process, gastrointestinal disorders, risk factors, and the like. The second includes sources that focus on diagnostic tests of disorders of the digestive system. The third focuses on the role of diet and nutrition in the prevention and treatment of gastrointestinal disorders.

If you want to know more about digestive disorders, the odds are that you will find a suitable source of information listed in the following pages.

Print
Materials

The publications listed here are either free or available for purchase. Not every available publication is included; rather, this list provides a representative selection of those print materials that constitute the best and most valuable publications available.

You may find some publications in your library or bookstore that are not listed here. Some are not included in these pages simply because they are not generally available. Some, perhaps, were published since this book was completed. Others, however, were reviewed and judged to be less useful than those that are cited in these pages.

Within each section, the publications are listed in alphabetical order by book or pamphlet title.

How to Obtain These Publications

The National Digestive Diseases Information Clearinghouse publications are available from the clearinghouse. Books published by general trade publishers can be found in libraries or ordered by your local bookstore. Where the publication is available only directly from the publisher, the address, phone number, and pertinent order information are included in the entry.

General Information

About Stomach Ulcers
Washington, D.C.: National Digestive Diseases Information
   Clearinghouse, 1987. 4 pages.
NIH Publication Number 87-676
Free

Following a brief discussion of the normal function of the stomach in the digestive process, the causes, associated risk factors, and symptoms of stomach ulcer are described. Diagnostic techniques and major methods of treatment, including the use of acid-inhibiting medications, diet, and surgery, are discussed.

Advice for the Patient, Volume II
Rockville, Maryland: The U.S. Pharmacopoeial Convention,
   Inc., 1985. 426 pages.
$23.95

Organized by generic name, this standard reference manual identifies the use and side effects of drugs and offers other information about over-the-counter and prescription medications.

It can be purchased from the U.S. Pharmacopeial Convention, Inc., 12601 Twinbrook Parkway, Rockville, Maryland 20852. Many libraries have this volume in their reference collection.

Age Page: Digestive Do's and Don'ts
Bethesda, Maryland: National Institute on Aging, 1986. 6 pages. Free

This fact sheet lists steps to maintain digestive health, describes digestive disorders common among older people, and offers suggestions for when to see the doctor.

It can be obtained by writing the National Institute on Aging, Building 31, Room 5C35, 9000 Rockville Pike, Bethesda, Maryland 20892.

Age Page: Smoking: It's Never Too Late to Stop
Bethesda, Maryland: National Institute on Aging, 1985. 2 pages. Free

This fact sheet provides basic information about what smoking does to your body and how to quit the habit. Information on how to contact support groups and other organizations in your area is presented.

A copy of this publication can be obtained by writing the National Institute on Aging, Building 31, Room 5C35, 9000 Rockville Pike, Bethesda, Maryland 20892.

Are You an Ulcer Person?
Los Angeles: Center for Ulcer Research and Education
    Foundation, 1985. 12 pages.
Free

The causes, symptoms, complications, and treatment of ulcers are discussed. Good basic information for the ulcer sufferer and his or her family is provided.

Bleeding in the Digestive Tract
Washington, D.C.: National Digestive Diseases Information
    Clearinghouse, 1986. 4 pages.
NIH Publication Number 87-1133
Free

This fact sheet explains that bleeding is a symptom of problems
in the digestive system rather than a disease in itself. It describes
the common digestive disorders that may give rise to bleeding
and how these disorders can be worsened by lifestyle factors such
as the use of certain drugs and smoking. Methods of diagnosis
and treatment of gastrointestinal problems, a glimpse at possible future treatments, and a glossary of common terms round
out the information provided.

Coping with Food Allergy
Frazier, Claude A., M.D.
New York, New York: Quadrangle/The New York Times Book
    Co., 1985. 278 pages.
$9.95

This book explains what a food allergy is and how it works,
and lists the foods that commonly cause symptoms. It points out
that food allergies can affect the gastrointestinal system, causing abdominal pain, recurrent diarrhea, and persistent constipation. An intriguing book for anyone with unexplained symptoms.

Diarrhea: Infectious and Other Causes
Washington, D.C.: National Digestive Diseases Information
    Clearinghouse, 1985. 4 pages.
NIH Publication Number 86-2749
Free

This fact sheet discusses one of the most common symptoms
associated with gastrointestinal disorders. The causes of this condition, why it is dangerous to some people, and what to do about
it are among the subjects presented.

Digestion: Fueling the System
Whitfield, Phillip
New York, New York: Torstar Books, 1985. 164 pages.
$19.95

Lavishly illustrated with large, detailed color plates on the structures and organs of digestion, this is a helpful book for anyone who has difficulty visualizing the relationship between components in the system.

Digestive Health and Disease: A Glossary
Washington, D.C.: National Digestive Diseases Information
   Clearinghouse, 1986. 12 pages.
NIH Publication Number 87-2750
Free

This book lists over 200 commonly used terms relating to digestive health and disease.

Facts & Fallacies About Digestive Diseases
Washington, D.C.: National Digestive Diseases Information
   Clearinghouse, 1986. 7 pages.
NIH Publication Number 86-2673
Free

Widely held but erroneous beliefs concerning hiatal hernia, ulcers, gallbladder disease, and pancreatitis, among other disorders, are explained and clarified in this helpful pamphlet.

Gallstone Disease
Washington, D.C.: National Digestive Diseases Information
   Clearinghouse, 1986. 4 pages.
Free

This easy-to-read fact sheet provides basic information on gallstone disease. Beginning with a brief discussion of the normal function of the gallbladder, it goes on to describe the processes involved in the formation of gallstones, including hereditary, environmental, and other risk factors. In addition to the classic symptoms associated with gallstones, information on diagnostic procedures, treatments, and outlook for the future is provided.

Gallstones and Other Gallbladder Disorders
Cedar Grove, New Jersey: American Liver Foundation, 1985.
    6 pages.
Free

This publication provides information on the gallbladder's function and the formation of gallstones.

A copy may be obtained by writing to the American Liver Foundation, 998 Pompton Avenue, Cedar Grove, New Jersey 07009, or by calling (800) 223-0179.

Gas in the Digestive Tract
Washington, D.C.: National Digestive Diseases Information
    Clearinghouse, 1985. 4 pages.
NIH Publication Number 85-883
Free

This informative fact sheet discusses the causes of belching and gas in the digestive system, the relation of gas to particular foods, and how gas can underlie certain types of abdominal pain and distension. Suggestions are offered for those who are troubled by this common condition.

Gastroenterology (3rd Edition)
Boicher, I.A. (Editor)
Philadelphia, Pennsylvania: Saunders, 1982. 388 pages.
$24.95

An excellent medical reference text for anyone who wants detailed information about any aspect of this subject.

Gastroenterology
Given, Barbara A., and Simmons, Sandra J.
St. Louis, Missouri: The C.V. Mosby Company, 1983. 528 pages.
$25.95

A standard medical reference for detailed information on the conditions and diseases of the digestive system, as well as current principles of care.

Gastrointestinal Disease: Pathophysiology & Diagnosis & Management (3rd Edition)
Sleisinger, M.H., and Fordtran, J.S.
Philadelphia, Pennsylvania: Saunders, 1983. 2 volumes.
$110.00
In print since 1947, this is a standard medical text and reference book. Although highly technical, it is comprehensive and authoritative.

Gastrointestinal Disorders
Nurses Clinical Library
Springhouse, Pennsylvania: Springhouse Corporation, 1985.
  192 pages.
$19.95

Written for nurses, this book provides an authoritative discussion of gastrointestinal disorders in somewhat less technical terms than standard medical reference works.

Heartburn
Washington, D.C.: National Digestive Diseases Information
  Clearinghouse, 1986. 4 pages.
NIH Publication Number 86-882
Free

Heartburn, one of the most commonly experienced digestive symptoms, is discussed in relation to problems of the lower esophageal sphincter, acid reflux, diet, and other factors. Self-help tips to control heartburn are provided, as well as discussions of possible complications, medical treatments, and the role of surgery.

Histamine Receptors
Yellin, Tobias O. (Editor)
Jamaica, New York: Spectrum Publishers, Inc., 1979. 418 pages.
$35.00

A highly technical reference text detailing the characteristics of histamine receptors in the body. Since use of histamine receptor antagonists is one form of acid-suppressing treatment of ulcers, this book provides more detailed information on the basis for the success of this therapy.

How to Stop Smoking: A Preventive Medicine Institute/Strang
  Clinic Health Action Plan
New York, New York: Holt, Rinehart and Winston, 1981.
  160 pages.
$12.95

This thoughtful publication from two prestigious organizations provides a systematic approach to permanent behavior change with regard to smoking. It is a simple step-by-step way to achieve this goal through self-assessment and easy-to-follow recommendations for change.

The Merck Manual of Diagnosis and Therapy
Merck, Sharp & Dohme Research Laboratories.
Rahway, New Jersey: Merck & Co., 1982.
  1600 pages.
$11.95

One of the most comprehensive and authoritative medical references available. Though fairly technical, it provides useful information on all aspects of diagnosis and treatment.

Peptic Ulcer: The Facts You Need to Know
Research Triangle Park, North Carolina: Glaxo, Inc., 1986.
    16 pages.
Free

   This informative booklet describes the causes, contributing factors, symptoms, diagnosis, and treatment of peptic disease.
   For a copy of this publication, write to Glaxo, Inc., Marketing Department, Five Moore Drive, Research Triangle Park, North Carolina 27709

Physician's Desk Reference
Oradell, New Jersey: Medical Economics Company, 1987.
    756 pages.
$36.95

   The PDR, as it is popularly known, is the standard reference book on thousands of prescription drugs available in the United States. Though intended primarily for physicians, the book is invaluable to anyone wanting information on drugs and related products. Information is indexed by manufacturer, product name, product classification, and generic and chemical name. One color-illustrated section is devoted to product identification. You may want to access this reference work in your library.

Physician's Desk Reference for Non-Prescription Drugs
    (8th Edition)
Oradell, New Jersey: Medical Economics Company, 1987.
    763 pages.
$21.95

   An excellent reference source on thousands of nonprescription drugs available in the United States. Information is clearly indexed. However, because the information is presented in technical terms, you may want to access this reference work in your library.

Smoking and Your Digestive System
Washington, D.C. National Digestive Diseases Information
   Clearinghouse, 1986. 4 pages.
NIH Publication Number 87-949
Free

The harmful effects of smoking on the digestive system, particularly its role in heartburn and ulcer, are described. The point
is clearly made that, no matter when you stop smoking, the liver
and other organs of the digestive system will benefit.

What Is Constipation?
Washington, D.C.: National Digestive Diseases Information
   Clearinghouse, 1986. 4 pages.
NIH Publication Number 87-2754
Free

This fact sheet provides definitions, causes, and other information about constipation. The effects this complaint has on
children and older people, the diagnostic tests used to determine
its causes, and the treatment available are discussed. Several common misconceptions are dispelled, and guidelines for avoiding
constipation are given.

What Is Hiatal Hernia?
Rosslyn, Virginia: National Digestive Diseases Information
   Clearinghouse, 1984. 2 pages.
Free

This fact sheet is crammed with information and diagrams
about one of the most common of all GI problems. The relationship between heartburn and hiatal hernia is explored, as well
as some of the complications that may be associated with this
condition.

What You Need to Know About Cancer of the Pancreas
Bethesda, Maryland: National Cancer Institute, 1986. 18 pages.
Free

This in-depth booklet describes cancer of the pancreas, its origins, treatments, and emotional aspects, and the direction of current research. An excellent source of information for the non-technical reader.

When Digestive Juices Corrode, You've Got an Ulcer
Rockville, Maryland: Food and Drug Administration, 1986.
  4 pages.
Free

A primer on the causes of ulcer disease and its treatment, including various drugs and surgical treatment techniques.

Your Digestive System and How It Works
Washington, D.C.: National Digestive Diseases Information
  Clearinghouse, 1986. 4 pages.
NIH Publication Number 86-2681
Free

The fundamentals of digestion, intestinal motility, the action of digestive juices, and the absorption of nutrients through the system are among the subjects covered in this fact sheet. The control of the digestive process by hormones and the action of nerve regulators are described in easy-to-understand language.

Diagnostic Tests

Diagnostic Tests for Digestive Disease: X-Rays and Ultrasound
Washington, D.C.: National Digestive Diseases Information
  Clearinghouse, 1986. 4 pages.
NIH Publication Number 87-887
Free

A brief but incisive overview of the role of X rays and ultrasound in the diagnosis of digestive problems. Explanation of "contrast studies," gallbladder X rays, arteriography, CT scanning, and ultrasound are provided in this helpful publication.

The Patient's Guide to Medical Tests
Pinckney, Cathy, and Pinckney, Edward, M.D.
New York, New York: Facts on File Publications, 1986.
  385 pages.
$12.95 (paperback); $21.95 (hardcover)

An excellent guide to more than 1,000 medical tests. Provides explanation of the reasons for doing the tests, the procedures and equipment used, the risk factors involved, and the ways the results are interpreted. A very useful book for the interested non-technical reader.

The People's Book of Medical Tests
Sobel, David, and Ferguson, Tom, M.D.
New York, New York: Summit Books, 1985. 509 pages.
$12.95 (paperback); $24.95 (hardcover)

A complete guide to more than 200 diagnostic and home medical tests. Gives information on costs, preparation, how long the test takes, whether or not it hurts, possible complications, and how the results may be useful.

Some Answers to Questions About Egd
Washington, D.C.: American Society for Gastrointestinal
  Endoscopy, 1985. 6 pages.
Free

One in the series of "Some Answers to . . ." brochures produced by the society, this booklet explains the purpose, procedures, and possible complications arising from esophagogastro-duodenoscopy (EGD).
  This brochure can be obtained by writing to the society at 13 Elm Street, Manchester, Massachusetts 01944.

Some Answers to Questions About ERCP
Washington, D.C.: American Society for Gastrointestinal
  Endoscopy, 1986. 6 pages.
Free

One in the series of "Some Answers to . . ." brochures produced by the society, this brochure explains the purpose of endoscopic retrograde cholangiopancreatography (ERCP), how the test is performed, and possible complications arising from the procedure.

This brochure can be obtained by writing to the society at 13 Elm Street, Manchester, Massachusetts 01944.

The X-Ray Information Book
Laws, Priscilla W., and The Public Citizen Health Research Group
New York, New York: Farrar, Straus, Giroux, 1983. 153 pages. $5.95

This information book puts into clear perspective the benefits and risks associated with medical X rays. It offers practical suggestions on how to avoid unnecessary exposure and discusses alternatives to X rays.

Diet and Nutrition

Age Page: Nutrition—A Lifelong Concern
Bethesda, Maryland: National Institute on Aging, 1987. 2 pages. Free

This fact sheet provides basic nutritional information, including facts about the benefits of dietary fiber. Particularly appropriate for readers in middle age and beyond.

A copy can be obtained by writing the National Institute on Aging, Building 31, Room 5C35, 9000 Rockville Pike, Bethesda, Maryland 20892.

All About Fat and Cancer Risk
Falls Church, Virginia: American Institute for Cancer Research, 1986. 16 pages.
Free

This booklet provides a great deal of helpful information, including the relationship between a diet high in fat and the risk of developing cancer.

To obtain a copy, write to the American Institute for Cancer Research, 500 N. Washington Street, Suite 100, Falls Church, Virginia 22046.

Fiber in Human Nutrition
Spiller, G.A., and Amen, R.J. (Editors)
New York, New York: Plenum Press, 1976. 278 pages.
$35.00

This book, which incorporates varied and divergent contributions from numerous scientists, examines research on claims that plant fiber has positive effects on maintaining gastrointestinal health. An excellent sourcebook for anyone wanting an in-depth understanding of fiber and its effect on digestive functioning.

The Gallbladder Diet
Cedar Grove, New Jersey: American Liver Foundation, 1985.
    6 pages.
Free

This publication provides a dietary plan for patients who have gallbladder and biliary tract disease.

A copy may be obtained by writing to the American Liver Foundation, 998 Pompton Avenue, Cedar Grove, New Jersey 07009, or by calling (800) 223-0179.

Menus and Recipes to Lower Cancer Risk
Falls Church, Virginia: American Institute for Cancer Research,
    1985. 31 pages.
Free

The contribution that food can make to reducing the risk of cancer is discussed. Hints for controlling fat intake, along with menus and recipes, are provided.

To obtain a copy, write to the American Institute for Cancer Research, 500 N. Washington Street, Suite 100, Falls Church, Virginia 22046.

Nutrition in Health and Disease (17th Edition)
Anderson, L., Dibble, M.V., et al. (Editors)
Philadelphia, Pennsylvania, 1982. 794 pages.
$26.50

A reference text providing detailed information on carbohydrates, fats, proteins, water and electrolyte metabolism, nutrient utilization, and other aspects of nutrition. The book also provides information on diet in the care of various gastrointestinal diseases.

Audiovisual Materials

This section presents audiovisual materials recommended for patient and professional use. The materials are listed in alphabetical order by title and are divided into the same subject divisions used earlier: "General Information," "Diagnostic Tests," and "Diet and Nutrition."

Should you be unable to find relevant audiovisual materials listed in the following pages, write to the Digestive Diseases Clearinghouse, 1555 Wilson Boulevard, Suite 600, Rosslyn, Virginia 22209-2461 and request a copy of the Audiovisual Catalog of the Digestive Diseases Clearinghouse. That publication lists hundreds of videocassettes and films for both the patient and the medical professional.

Many public, professional, and medical libraries will have some of these materials for rental. Check with the reference librarian at your local library to help you find the nearest source.

General Information

Alcohol and the Liver
Available from: PBS Video
475 L'Enfant Plaza, S.W.
Washington, D.C. 20024
(800) 424-7963
29 minutes, color, 1978

Explains the effect of alcohol on the liver, including nutrition, toxicity, and death statistics.
Write for pricing information.

Common Disorders of the Swallowing Mechanism
Available from: National Audiovisual Center
Government Services Administration Order Section RL
Washington, D.C. 20409
(301) 763-1896
17 minutes, color, 1980
$85.00

This video provides one of the few detailed discussions of this subject for nontechnical viewers. It explains the processes that normally occur during swallowing. Then, through the use of fiberoptic endoscopy, it demonstrates many of the common disorders that can affect the swallowing mechanism.

Controlling Heartburn
Available from: American College of Physicians
Mary Bieter
4200 Pine Street
Philadelphia, Pennsylvania 19104
10 minutes, color, 1982
$175.00

The basic symptoms and causes of heartburn, one of the most commonly reported digestive complaints, are discussed. Stressing self-help, the program elaborates the various ways in which sufferers can control heartburn.

Digestive System
Available from: University of Wisconsin
Bureau of Audiovisual Instruction
University of Wisconsin
P.O. Box 2093
Madison, Wisconsin 53701
17 minutes, color, 1979
$13.50

The complex process of human digestion is clarified through the use of animation and laboratory research techniques, including remarkable scenes of digestive sequences filmed by X-ray motion picture photography. It provides a good understanding of what happens when food goes through the digestive system.

The Digestive System
Available from: University of Illinois
1325 South Oak Street
Champaign, Illinois 61620
19 minutes, color, 1981
$12.00

This program familiarizes the viewer with the "geography" of the digestive system by use of color animation and X-ray footage. The location and functions of the major components of the digestive system are introduced and explained, beginning with the salivary glands. Intended for use by the public, this program includes a description of various digestive enzymes and chemicals and the nutritional elements needed for a balanced diet. The contribution of each of these components to the overall function of the digestive system is explained.

*Free Yourself from Digestive Pain: A Guide to Preventing and
    Curing Your Digestive Illness*
(RD23961)
Available on loan free to blind or physically disabled individuals
    from: Library of Congress
National Library for the Blind and Physically Disabled
1291 Taylor Street, N.W.
Washington, D.C. 20542
(202) 287-5100

Reviews various maladies of the digestive system. Each chapter focuses on a specific problem, delving into the cause, the course of the ailment, and the treatment. Among topics discussed are acid indigestion, ulcers, heartburn, intestinal gas, and hemorrhoids.

Gallbladder Disease
Available from: PBS Video
475 L'Enfant Plaza, S.W.
Washington, D.C. 20024
(800) 424-7963
29 minutes, color, 1978
$175.00

This problem explains the function of the gallbladder in the digestive process, why gallstones form, and the surgical procedures used to remove them.

Heartburn
Available from: NIADDK-NIH
Annex Building
Room 3A17A—Ms. Billie Mackey
Bethesda, Maryland 20205
5 minutes, color, 1982
$40.00

A leading medical expert discusses the common cause and symptoms of heartburn and explains various methods by which it can be treated effectively.

Heartburn and Hiatal Health
Available from: PBS Video
475 L'Enfant Plaza, S.W.
Washington, D.C. 20024
(800) 424-7963
29 minutes, color, 1982
Rental: $55.00   Sale: $200.00

Two prominent doctors from the University of Texas Health
Science Center discuss the common complaint of heartburn and
the problem of hiatal hernia. Sufferers from these conditions and
other general viewers will find the conversation interesting and
informative.

I Am Joe's Stomach
Available from: Pyramid Films
Box 1048
Santa Monica, California 90406
25 minutes, color, 1975
Rental: $50.00

An excellent film that uses live action sequences and
three-dimensional animation to illustrate the digestive process in
the stomach. The activities of the secretory glands and their functions are explained. The potentially harmful effects of overeating,
stress, and overmedication are also discussed.

Jane Brody's The New York Times Guide to Personal Health
   (RC-21343)
Available on loan free to blind or physically disabled individuals
   from: Library of Congress
National Library for the Blind and Physically Disabled
1291 Taylor Street, N.W.
Washington, D.C. 20542
(202) 287-5100
6 audiocassettes, 1971

Collection of the author's "Personal Health" columns on
physical health and emotional fitness. The essays are arranged

by topic under such categories as nutrition, exercise, sexuality, drugs, and emotional health. The focus is away from heroic therapies for disease and toward individual responsibility for health.

Living with Your Ulcer (RC 16441)
Available on loan free to blind or physically disabled individuals
    from: Library of Congress
National Library for the Blind and Physically Disabled
1291 Taylor Street, N.W.
Washington, D.C. 20542
(202) 287-5100
Audiocassette, 1971
Berlund, Theodore, and Spellburg, Mitchell

A guide for ulcer patients and their families about the causes, symptoms, diagnosis, and treatment of ulcers. Includes menus and recipes.

Peptic Ulcer
Available from: National Institutes of Health
Office of Clinical Reports and Inquiries
Building 10, Room 5C 305
Bethesda, Maryland 20205
(301) 496-6158
60 minutes, color, 1980
$20.00

The underlying causes as well as the prevalence of ulcers in the modern world are described in detail. The differences between gastric and duodenal ulcers and their symptoms, diagnosis, and treatment are presented. The film shows the layperson what can be done about this widespread health problem.

Peptic Ulcer
Available from: Milner Fenwick
2125 Greenspring Drive
Timonium, Maryland 21093
(800) 638-8652
12 minutes, color, 1982
$250.00

This video program is designed to give sufferers of peptic ulcer a comprehensive picture of the classic symptoms associated with this common disorder. Emphasis is placed on the importance of accurate diagnosis. The program also explains appropriate therapy to relieve pain, prevent recurrences, and avoid complications. This program is currently being revised and updated.

Peptic Ulcer
Available from: Professional Research, Inc.
930 Pitner
Evanston, Illinois 60202
(800) 421-2363
15 minutes, color, 1984
Rental: $55.00   Sale: $295.00

The process involved in the formation of ulcers, the factors that worsen or heal them, and other aspects of ulcers are discussed. Stresses the patient's responsibility for contributing to treatment by following the doctor's recommendations regarding medication, rest, and diet.

Peptic Ulcer Surgery Series: Before and After Surgery
Available from: Scene II Productions, Inc.
22 Front Street West, 8th Floor
Toronto, Canada M5J IC4
19 minutes, color, 1980
$395.00

Designed for patients who may be undergoing surgery for ulcers, this video program outlines what to expect upon admission to the hospital and what surgery for ulcers entails.

The Sensitive Stomach
Available from: Time-Life Film, Inc.
1271 Avenue of the Americas
New York, New York 10019
15 minutes, color, 1979

This self-help video portrays how simple and complex gastrointestinal disorders can be avoided and controlled. Among the subjects discussed are why ulcers are so common, how to be sensible about diets, the dangers of overeating, and how to avoid nervous indigestion.
Write for pricing information.

Troubles in the Digestive Tract
Available from: Professional Research, Inc.
930 Pitner
Evanston, Illinois 60202
(800) 421-2363
10 minutes, color, 1984
Rental: $30.00   Sale: $295.00

This program is particularly helpful to parents and others working with children. It discusses disturbances that may arise within a child's digestive tract, including stool changes, constipation, diarrhea, and vomiting. It also explains the proper method for giving an enema.

Ulcers (RC 13568)
Available on loan free to blind or physically disabled individuals
    from: Library of Congress
National Library for the Blind and Physically Disabled

1291 Taylor Street, N.W.
Washington, D.C. 20542
(202) 287-5100
Audiocassette, 1978

An ulcer specialist answers questions about the disease and its treatment. He discusses who gets ulcers and why, and focuses on genetic, environmental, and psychological causes. Includes several methods for treatment, including surgery, drugs, and diet.

Zollinger–Ellison's Disease
Available from: Abbott Laboratories
A-V Services, Dept. 383
Abbott Park, Illinois 60064
(312) 937-3933
26 minutes, color, 1981
Rental: $15.00

This program is designed for use by physicians and provides one of the few available discussions of this condition available in the audiovisual medium. Though quite technical, the video discusses the syndrome in all its variations. The classical symptoms are described and related to tumors of the pancreas, which produce a gastrinlike substance. Those with special interest may arrange rental with the assistance of an understanding physician.

Diagnostic Tests

Bleeding in the Gut
Available from: NIADDK-NIH
Annex Building
Room 3A17A—Ms. Billie Mackey
Bethesda, Maryland 20205
5 minutes, color, 1982
$40.00

A leading medical expert discusses the causes of bleeding in the digestive tract and the diagnostic procedures commonly used to diagnose the underlying causes.

The Inside Story
Available from: The National Audiovisual Center
Government Services Administration
Order Section RL
Washington, D.C. 20409
(301) 763-1896
26 minutes, color, 1978
$126.00

This video program shows a medical student studying the upper GI endoscopy procedure. It is a particularly helpful film because the student's explanation of the procedure to an anxious patient makes the process clear to viewers with many of the same concerns and questions.

Upper GI Endoscopy
Available from: Milner Fenwick
2125 Greenspring Drive
Timonium, Maryland 21093
(800) 638-8652
8 minutes, color, 1982
$250.00

This program describes how the endoscopic procedure is used to identify and diagnose common problems in the upper digestive tract. It emphasizes the importance of proper preparation to obtain good results.

Diet and Nutrition

Basic Nutrition: Let's Make a Deal
Available from: Professional Research, Inc.
930 Pitner
Evanston, Illinois 60202
(800) 421-2363
10 minutes, color, 1984
Rental: $30.00   Sale: $295.00

This entertaining video program presents nutritional facts and fallacies in the form of a game show. It provides information on nutrients and how the body uses them; discusses calories, weight, diet, and disease; and provides guidelines for healthful nutrition and meal planning.

The Bland-Diet Cookbook (RC 15356)
Available on loan free to blind or physically disabled individuals
  from: Library of Congress
National Library for the Blind and Physically Disabled
1291 Taylor Street, N.W.
Washington, D.C. 20542
(202) 287-5100
Audiocassette, 1978

Offers more than 200 palatable recipes using soothing, mild foods for soups, sauces, salads, main dishes, and desserts. Menus for ulcer sufferers and low-residue and low-fat diets are also included.

The Body Works: Digestion
Available from: University of Illinois
1325 South Oak Street
Champaign, Illinois 61820
(800) 252-1359
27 minutes, color, 1979
Rental: $13.50

This program, produced by the Harvard Medical School, uses fiber optics, ultrasound, and anatomical models to show how the body gets the nutrients it needs from food and what the approximate "size" of the digestive system would be if "unrolled." Intended for a lay audience, the program enumerates and explains many of the functions of the liver.

Food, Energy and You
Available from: Professional Research, Inc.
930 Pitner
Evanston, Illinois 60202
(800) 421-2363
20 minutes, color, 1984
Rental: $38.00   Sale: $375.00

This film provides a clear, concise picture of how energy is used by our bodies and where it comes from in the foods we eat. The importance of getting a sufficient amount of food energy to maintain growth and development is shown.

Foods That Fight Cancer: A Diet and Vitamins Program That Protects the Entire Family (RC 20802)
Available on loan free to blind or physically disabled individuals from: Library of Congress
National Library for the Blind and Physically Disabled
1291 Taylor Street, N.W.
Washington, D.C. 20542
(202) 287-5100
2 audiocassettes, 1983

Easy-to-follow program for improving nutritional habits in accordance with the National Academy of Sciences report outlining links between diet and cancer. Shows how such specific foods as fruits and vegetables rich in vitamins A and C eaten daily may prevent some of the most common cancers.

Positive Approaches to Nutrition
Available from: Spectrum Films
2785 Roosevelt Street
Carlsbad, California 92008
20 minutes, color, 1984
Rental: $65.00   Preview: $35.00

This self-help video focuses on helping the viewer to make positive practical choices of food consumed at breakfast, lunch, and dinner. The program points out that important health benefits can be obtained if foods are consciously selected for their nutritional value.

What's Good to Eat?
Available from: Professional Research, Inc.
930 Pitner
Evanston, Illinois 60202
(800) 421-2363
20 minutes, color, 1984
Rental: $29.00   Sale: $320.00

This film is designed to give students an understanding of how the body uses nutrients from food and how food groups provide a useful guide for making reasonable choices. An overview of the basic nutritional components is provided. Proteins, vitamins, carbohydrates, fats, and minerals are all explained and related to everyday foods.

Your Diet: Fiber
Available from: Professional Research, Inc.
930 Pitner
Evanston, Illinois 60202
(800) 421-2363
13 minutes, color, 1984
Rental: $30.00   Sale: $295.00

The role of fiber in a healthful diet is discussed. The program also provides information on the best sources of fiber among the foods we commonly eat.

INDEX

Abbott Laboratories, 133
About Stomach Ulcers, 112
Abscess, 48, 51
Achalasia (cardio-spasm), 18–19;
esophageal cancer and, 20;
severity of, 18; symptoms of,
18; treatment for, 18–19; typical
sufferer of, 18
Acid-inhibiting drugs, 84–85;
anti-cholinergics, 85; H2
blockers, 84–85;
metoclopramide, 85
Acid neutralizers: *See* Antacids
Acute Cholecystitis: *See*
Cholecystitis, acute
Acute duodenal erosions: *See*
Duodenal erosions, acute
Acute gastric erosions: *See*
Gastric erosions, acute
Acute gastritis: *See* Gastritis,
acute
Acute pancreatitis: *See*
Pancreatitis, acute
Acute stress ulcers: *See* Duodenal
erosions, acute; Gastric
erosions, acute
Advice for the Patient, Volume II,
112–113
*Age Page: Digestive Do's and
Don'ts*, 113
*Age Page: Nutrition—A Lifelong
Concern*, 123
*Age Page: Smoking: It's Never
Too Late to Stop*, 113
Alcohol abuse: acute gastritis
and, 22; acute pancreatitis and,
47; audiovisual material
concerning, 126; chronic
pancreatitis and, 50; esophageal
cancer and, 20; organizations
concerning, 102–103

Alcohol and the Liver
(audiovisual material), 126
Alkali, 6
All About Fat and Cancer Risk,
123–124
American Cancer Society, 98
American College of Physicians,
126
American Diabetes Association,
Inc., 98–99
American Dietetic Association,
99
American Digestive Disease
Society, 99
American Heart Association,
Inc., 100
American Institute for Cancer
Research, 123, 124, 125
American Liver Foundation, 116,
124
American Medical Association,
100
American Pharmaceutical
Association, 100–101
American Society for
Gastrointestinal Endoscopy,
122, 123
Amphojel, 81–83
Anemia, pernicious: atrophic
gastritis and, 35, 36; vitamin B-
12 absorption test for, 75
Anesthesiologist, 96
Antacids (acid neutralizers), 81–
83; duodenal ulcers and, 43–44
Antiarthritis medicines: acute
gastritis and, 23
Anticholinergics, 85
Antispasmodic drugs (muscle
relaxants), 83–84
Antrectomy: *See* Gastrectomy
Are You an Ulcer Person?, 113

139